Native American Herbalist's Bible

14 Books in 1

The Complete Guide with 600+ Herbal Medicines & Plant Remedies. Improve Your Life-Long Vitality by Your Own Herbal Dispensatory and Apothecary Table

Amayeta Narayan

© Copyright 2022 - All rights reserved.

The content contained within this book may not be reproduced, duplicated or transmitted without direct written permission from the author or the publisher. Under no circumstances will any blame or legal responsibility be held against the publisher, or author, for any damages, reparation, or monetary loss due to the information contained within this book. Either **directly or indirectly.**

Legal Notice:
This book is copyright protected. This book is only for personal use. You cannot amend, distribute, sell, use, quote or paraphrase any part, or the content within this book, without the consent of the author or publisher.

Disclaimer Notice:
Please note the information contained within this document is for educational and entertainment purposes only. All effort has been executed to present accurate, up to date, and reliable, complete information. No warranties of any kind are declared or implied. Readers acknowledge that the author is not engaging in the rendering of legal, financial, medical or professional advice. The content within this book has been derived from various sources. Please consult a licensed professional before attempting any techniques outlined in this book.

By reading this document, the reader agrees that under no circumstances is the author responsible for any losses, direct or indirect, which are incurred as a result of the use of information contained within this document, including, but not limited to, errors, omissions, or inaccuracies.

Contents

BOOK 1: INTRODUCTION TO NATIVE AMERICAN 6
- Chapter 1: History And Origins 7
- Chapter 2: Native Americans And Their Connection With Nature 9
- Chapter 3: The Fundamental Values Of Native American People 13
- Chapter 4: Herbalism History 15
- Chapter 5: Herbalism And Modern Medicine 17

BOOK 2: NATIVE AMERICAN HERBAL REMEDIES 19
- Chapter 1: Historical Overview Of Herbalism 20
- Chapter 2: Common Diseases Treatable With Herbs 20

BOOK 3: NATIVE AMERICAN HERBALISM ENCYCLOPEDIA VOL 1 27
- Chapter 1: The Bases Of Native American Herbalism 28
- Chapter 2: The Best 200 Medical Herbs To Use 29

BOOK 4: NATIVE AMERICAN HERBALISM ENCYCLOPEDIA VOL 2 48
- Chapter 1: The Best 200 Medical Herbs To Use 49

BOOK 5: NATIVE AMERICAN ESSENTIAL OILS VOL 1 69
- Chapter 1: An Overview Of Essential Oils 70
- Chapter 2: The Benefits Of Using Oils 71
- Chapter 3: How To Use Essential Oils 73
- Chapter 4: How To Store Essential Oils 75

BOOK 6: NATIVE AMERICAN ESSENTIAL OILS VOL 2 77
- Chapter 1: List Of All Crucial Essential Oils 78

BOOK 7: NATIVE AMERICAN SPIRITUALITY 81

    Chapter 1: Native Americans Beliefs And Practices 82

    Chapter 2: Native Americans Spirituality In Medicines 85

BOOK 8: NATIVE AMERICAN NATURAL MEDICINE 88

    Chapter 1: The Cherokee Legend 89

    Chapter 2: Sacred Medicines For Native Americans 90

    Chapter 3: Main Native Americans Medicinal Plants 93

BOOK 9: NATIVE AMERICAN STONES & CRYSTALS 96

    Chapter 1: Basic Things To Know About Healing Stones And Crystals 97

    Chapter 2: Most Used Crystals And Stones 100

BOOK 10: NATIVE AMERICAN HERBAL GARDENING 104

    Chapter 1: Gardening And Herbalist Tools To Have 105

    Chapter 2: The Two Types Of Beginner-Friendly Gardens 110

    Chapter 3: The Process Of Preparation And Planting Your Herbs 114

    Chapter 4: Tips On How To Grow Herbs In Your Garden 116

BOOK 11: HERBAL RECIPES FOR YOUR CHILD'S HEALTH 119

    Chapter 1: Common Medicinal Herbs And Their Properties 120

    Chapter 2: The Best Medical Herbs For Kids 122

    Chapter 3: Homemade Herbs Recipes For Kid's Health 124

BOOK 12: NATIVE AMERICANS DO IT YOURSELF 126

    Chapter 1: Infusions 127

    Chapter 2: Tea 128

    Chapter 3: Decoction 129

    Chapter 4: Popsicles 130

Chapter 5: Baths 130

Chapter 6: Washcloths 131

BOOK 13: NATIVE AMERICAN DISPENSATORY 134

Chapter 1: Native American Medicine 135

Chapter 2: Extraction Process 140

Chapter 3: Different Ways Of Preparing And Using Your Herbs 143

Chapter 4: The Process Of Storing Your Herbs 148

BOOK 14: NATIVE AMERICAN MEDICINAL PLANTS 151

Chapter 1: Plants For Beauty 152

Chapter 2: Plants For Healing 153

Chapter 3: Plants For Fertility 154

Chapter 4: Plants For Wealth 155

Chapter 5: Plants For Good Luck 156

Chapter 6: Plants For Protection 158

CONCLUSION 160

Book 1: Introduction To Native American

Chapter 1: History And Origins

Native Americans are one of North America's most fascinating and visible minority groups. Their history stretches back thousands of years, and their culture is alive and well today. In this section post, we will explore the origins of Native Americans and their relationship to the land. We will also look at some of the critical events in their history, from the arrival of the Europeans to the present day. Knowledge is power, and understanding Native American culture and history is an important part of empowering yourself as a member of this minority group.

The Pre-Columbian Era

The Pre-Columbian Era spans roughly before Columbus sailed to America in 1492. This era is marked by the development of civilizations in Mesoamerica, South America, and North America. The cultures of the Pre-Columbian Era were diverse and complex, with many traditions and beliefs that have since disappeared.

Mesoamerica was the most densely populated region of the Americas before Columbus's arrival. The Maya Civilization was one of the most advanced pre-Columbian societies, with a well-developed system of hieroglyphics, a calendar, and a writing system called Coptic. The Aztec Empire was another powerful Mesoamerican society with a strong military and political presence.

South America was home to many different cultures during the Pre-Columbian Era. The Inca Empire was one of the most powerful societies in South America, with an extensive network of roads and buildings. The Mayans also had a significant presence in South America, building some of the world's largest pyramids.

North America was sparsely populated during the Pre-Columbian era, with only a few small settlements scattered across the continent. The indigenous people of North America were diverse and included members of several different cultures. The Navajo Nation is one example of an indigenous group that continues to live in North America today.

The Conquest of America by Spain

The Spanish conquest of America was a lengthy and brutal process that began in the late 15th century and ended centuries later with the arrival of the United States. The Spanish were, after all, conquering a continent with dozens of different cultures spread across it. They faced many challenges in their attempt to take control, including fierce resistance from the Native American people. In the end, Spain conquered most of what is now known as America, but there were tens of millions of casualties.

The Indigenous Peoples Who Inhabited America before European Colonization

The Indigenous Peoples who inhabited America before European colonization are the Paleo-Indians. These people ranged in age and culture from the oldest human remains found in North America, which date back to over 15,000 years ago, to the highly mobile hunter-gatherers of the Great Lakes region. By 1000 BC, however, most Native American groups had developed semi-sedentary cultures based around villages, and villages were beginning to form permanent settlements.

The first Europeans to arrive in the United States were the Norsemen in the ninth century AD. They explored both coasts of present-day North America before settling in Newfoundland. From there, they began an exploration of inland regions, meeting and trading with various Native American groups. In 1492, Christopher Columbus landed on what he thought was an island off the coast of Cuba. He soon after claimed the entire Western Hemisphere for Spain.

Spain's interest in acquiring territory in North America grew as they saw increasing competition from France to control Europe's maritime trade routes. In 1513, Spanish explorer Francisco Vásquez de Coronado set out from Mexico City with a large entourage seeking gold and indigenous slaves. Instead, he discovered a vast landscape of rugged mountains and wide open plains that he named New Mexico. De Coronado's expedition continued westward through Arizona and into California, where he met his death at the hands of native Americans near modern-day Sacramento.

In 1542 another Spanish expedition led by Hernando de Soto explored much of what is now the southeastern United States. De Soto's expedition was marked by violence and destruction as he attempted to subjugate the native populations and pillage their resources. In 1580, Juan Ponce de León claimed Florida for Spain. In 1584, a group of Spanish soldiers led by Pedro Menéndez de Avilés sailed up the east coast of Florida, searching for a route to the Pacific Ocean.

In 1585, Menéndez de Avilés founded St. Augustine, the first European settlement in what would become Florida. By 1600, France had emerged as Spain's primary rival in North America and began to invest more resources into exploration and conquest. In 1607, King James I of England granted a charter to the Massachusetts Bay Colony, leading to hundreds of English Puritans arriving in what is now Massachusetts.

In 1614, a Dutch expedition led by Hendrick Corstiaensen discovered New York City while exploring along the Hudson River. The next year, a group of Englishmen led by Captain John Smith explored both sides of the Appalachian Mountains, which would later be named for them. In 1618, French explorer Samuel de Champlain founded Quebec City, which became the first European settlement in what is now the United States.

In 1620, Spanish explorer Hernando de Soto led a second expedition into Florida, which resulted in the enslavement of thousands of Native Americans. In 1624, Englishman Captain John Smith founded Jamestown, the first permanent English settlement in North America. From 1626 to 1628, Dutch explorers Jacob Leisler and Willem Verhulst explored what is now Maine.

In 1630, Englishman Roger Williams founded Providence, Rhode Island, which refused to accept Protestantism as the state religion. In 1632, French explorer Samuel de Champlain founded Port Royal on South Carolina's Ashley River, which soon became a major trade center for fur traders. In 1634, Englishman Sir Walter Raleigh established the first English colony in North America on Roanoke Island in North Carolina. Still, it was abandoned less than two years later.

In 1636-37, Dutch explorer Adriaen Block led an expedition up the Hudson River, resulting in the founding of Albany and Yonkers by Dutch settlers. In 1638, Massachusetts Bay Colony Governor John Winthrop proclaimed that all British subjects must live independently.

The Early History of the Native American People

It is difficult to determine when the first people migrated to North America. Still, they did so at some point in prehistoric times. Archeological evidence indicates that early inhabitants of the continent were hunter-gatherers and that by 8000 BC, agriculture had begun to be practiced. By 3000 BC, groups of nomadic hunter-gatherers had begun settling down in certain areas and developing intricate spiritual beliefs and practices. The first settlements were located along the Atlantic seaboard. Still, as the continent was explored more and more, people began moving into new parts of the country. By 1000 AD, many tribes had been established throughout the United States.

The cultures of the various tribes varied greatly from region to region, with some being much more advanced than others. While many tribes shared similar religious beliefs and ceremonies, each tribe maintained unique traditions and customs. One of the most important aspects of Native American culture was its oral tradition, which consisted of stories and legends passed down from generation to generation. These stories served as a source of wisdom for the tribal members and anyone. They wished to learn about traditional customs and beliefs.

Despite their diverse cultures and languages, all Native Americans shared a common ancestry and history. They were physically similar to people living in Europe or Asia Minor, indicating that they likely originated in one or more distant regions. It is uncertain what caused these people.

Humans crossed the Bering land bridge from Asia into Alaska centuries ago, during the end of the Ice Age. North American shoreline was explored by their ancestors. They had already occupied practically the whole continent by 1000 BC. Exactly when the earliest inhabitants of the Americas arrived is a mystery.

Americans have a rich cultural heritage because of their long history of migration, which has seen them cultivate several languages, traditions, and civilizations all across the world for millennia. As in Europe, Africa, and Asia, the Americas have as many distinct tribal nations as other continents.

Some Indigenous American tribes began experimenting with new crops due to shifting climates and burgeoning populations. Others stayed in the area and developed and became very adept farmers. Corn and squash were farmed by Mexican Indians as far back as 5 500 BC. Deer and bison were hunted and reared as food for the family. They burnt off areas of land regularly to provide grass for the animals. Many coastal cultures used practical tactics to catch fish and hunt marine creatures from boats.

Several Native American states with populations in the tens of thousands arose after 2000 BC. They built a network of trading channels that stretched throughout the globe.

In 1492, Columbus sailed to the "New World" and launched the European colonization of the Americas. Smallpox and measles were among the illnesses introduced by the Europeans. Native Americans were immediately infected with these new illnesses. Many native cities were decimated by the invasion.

Europe's expanding population needed new farmland and employment, so the Europeans set out to colonize America. They frequently had to engage in land wars with Native American tribes to do this. The Europeans had an edge in these confrontations due to various circumstances. While some Native American tribes fought back against colonialism, many were finally compelled to give up their country.

Today The number of Native Americans living in North America and Europe is increasing again. There has been a significant increase in political success for Native American leaders in the battle for their people. In addition, governments and others have become more aware of the need to respect indigenous cultures and traditions while responding to the needs of Native Americans.

Native Americans are often mentioned in histories of health, disease, and medicine in the United States, particularly in the imperial and early republican periods. While illness outbreaks are often mentioned in the history of Native American civilizations and early European encounters, there is little emphasis on wellness and healing in this context.

Medicinal plants indigenous to the United States, Alaska, and Hawaii have been used for centuries by Native American, Alaskan Native, and Hawaiian healers for various ailments. Many herbal medicines and their uses may be found throughout many cultures.

Before the arrival of Europeans, Native Americans relied heavily on indigenous plants for food and medicine. Current attempts to enhance current generations' diets are centered on indigenous flora. With indigenous foods, Hawai i's Waianae and Captain Cook diets strive to limit fat, calories, and additives while increasing the nutritional value of the island's food supply to improve health. Native Alaskans and other Indian tribes are working together to promote the preservation of indigenous meals. Food, in this sense, is medicine in the truest meaning of the word.

Chapter 2: Native Americans And Their Connection With Nature

Nature's importance in Native American culture has been thoroughly documented throughout history and continues to be so now. Religion, everyday rituals, mythology, literature, cuisine, medicine, art, and many other aspects of American Indian culture are all influenced by the natural environment. Their way of life is intrinsically linked to the land and the environment.

It's easy to see how and why nature has become so important in all forms of Native American culture once you understand the crucial function it plays in their society. We've posted a brief but comprehensive description of how nature shapes and defines indigenous peoples' worldviews. This material is an instructive and practical way to immerse yourself in the fascinating world of Native American art and genuinely enjoy it.

Native Americans Have A Deep Appreciation For The Natural World

In American Indian culture, nature is cherished above all else. The concept is intricately related to society's spiritual beliefs, both of which serve as important identifying characteristics of its perspective and way of life.

Native Americans believe that all items and aspects of the Earth, both living and nonliving, have a distinct spirit that is part of the greater soul of the universe. This concept is related to Animism, a religion characterized by believing in and worshiping an underlying spirituality.

Animism theories embrace all living and natural items and nonliving occurrences. This category includes humans, plants, animals, elements, and geographical features such as a river, mountains, or thunderstorms. Native American culture appears to value and appreciate the land's essence and everything it provides.

There Is No Science Involved In Cultural Evolution

While there are numerous contradictory legends and conversations regarding the Earth's origins, science is usually the discipline used to explain how the cosmos works and how certain realities occur. Although the mechanism of photosynthesis is now a well-known and widely accepted explanation for plant development, to Native Americans, a growing flower was a gift from a land gifted with its own spirit.

Many American Indians, both in the past and now, looked to nature to interpret occurrences they couldn't fully comprehend. They believed that spirits dominated the Earth and its natural components. As a result, they began to worship, among other things, the wind, animals, plants, and water.

All Native American traditions agree that life is sacred and emanates from the soil, meaning Mother Earth is divine. This concept pervades every piece of work they produce.

Nature's Elements Have A Larger Significance

Nature traits are symbolic and multi-functional in the American Indian universe, making them valuable and pervasive in everything they accomplish and develop. Totems are used by Native Americans to achieve power and strength, and symbols are used in their writings and artwork to understand and connect with the rest of the world. If symbols symbolize their language, nature is the lexicon.

Trees, for example, are more than just a sign of life and healing; they also represent permanence and longevity. Distinct types play different roles. The Cherry tree is associated with rebirth and compassion; it promotes digestion, whereas the Elm is associated with developing wisdom and willpower. It can also be used to treat wounds.

An Animal Spirit is another example of how nature is intricately linked to Native American beliefs and traditions. Individuals frequently connect with a spirit animal—a guide who significantly influences who they are or how they live. Similar to Tribe Totems, organizations commonly select Spirit Creatures to serve as Tribe Totems, the most influential and prevalent animals in each tribe's region, and provide crucial resources and spiritual revelations to help people navigate life.

The Bat, for example, is the protector of the night, representing death and rebirth. In contrast, the Turtle guards Mother Earth and signifies persistence. The Pathfinder is the Wolf who leads with wisdom and a spirit of leadership. In Native American tradition, nature is the basic anchor for generating all spirit and life. Native American artists' representation of this worldview through art distinguishes them from their contemporaries. It helps their work to reach a wider audience. Understanding the significance of nature in their culture permits spectators to appreciate and comprehend the substantial, one-of-a-kind works created by American Indian artists.

Despite living in separate locations in what is now the United States, many different Native American tribes shared a pearl of comparable collective wisdom. They recognized and understood the interdependence of all ecological components. Humans, rocks, plants, and even animals depended on one another for survival and the health of their biological niche.

Everything we do as people has an impact on our environment. This basic concept equated Native Americans with the animals they hunted for food and the berries they gathered from the bush.

They were aware that their acts were having an effect. Because of this awareness, they regarded nature with a level of love and adoration that is sometimes ignored in modern society.

That doesn't mean you can't go deer hunting. It means that they hunted there after the baby season in the fall, thanking and respecting the animal for its gift to their life.

Native Americans altered their ecological niches to some extent. They cleared ground to make way for houses and fields. These changes were minimal, and as the tribe moved to a new location, the land quickly recovered. Archaeological digs have revealed remnants of their villages, although the sites have not harmed the ecosystem.

This technique of engaging with nature caused many issues when European settlers invaded America with very different land management practices. The Pilgrims and other early immigrants envisioned America as a land to conquer. Their writings and letters were frequently filled with fear of this strange new world and its inhabitants.

Native Americans, Whites, and Americans of varied cultural origins strive to reintroduce traditional earth management techniques. We consider the environment when we perceive ourselves as part of the system. Blaming others - politicians, foreign countries, the average citizen - is a popular political response.

We won't get very far blaming others. To transcend the blame game and even find a way to coexist with nature, we must all rise to the occasion and collaborate.

Self-Restraint

Many Native American tribes have a unique concept of self-control. The concept of self-control derives from community life and living together in the natural world, which may bring about unanticipated changes. Self-control is good when group strength is equated with survival in a communal culture.

Native peoples protected future generations' lives by limiting their use of natural resources. They left a legacy for future generations to carry on. They did not slaughter the planet for personal gain.

The Iroquois Confederacy's Seventh Generation doctrine "mandates that tribe decision-makers examine the ramifications of their acts and decisions for descendants seven generations into the future."

The Haudenosaunee Confederacy's government dates back to 1142 AD. Still, it was admired by Benjamin Franklin, who modeled aspects of the Constitution all upon its ideas. This is a network. Understand the links between animals, humans, and the environment that affects our lives and the lives of future generations

Changes In The Climate

Climate change appears to be a massive issue that affects everyone on the earth. Many American communities are looking to Native American knowledge to deal with these challenges.

Climate change has decimated Louisiana's Gulf Coast's coastal areas, as the Houma Nation experienced. Deliberate ecosystem devastation includes erosion, oil-industry harm, and the planned destruction of an ecosystem. They've spent decades living in the marshes and along the shore, subsisting on fishing, shrimping, and other subsistence activities.

As a result of climate change and industrialization, massive erosion has occurred along the Louisiana coast. The landscape has quickly changed, islands have vanished, and pollution has killed fish and crabs. The Houma will be unable to pass on their way of life to future generations since it has been destroyed.

Many fish and crustacean species breed in coastal marshlands. Indigenous coastal tribes have long preserved these environments by planting marsh meadows and trees.

As a result of this natural cycle, (baby fish) fry thrived. Several times, oil companies and commercial fisheries have built canals across these places, destroying this unique stream and significantly decreasing fish reproduction.

Agriculture

Native Americans are not widely regarded as the first farmers. A stereotype depicts the brave on a horse and living in a tent on the Great Plains.

However, according to popular belief, the first Native Americans came into touch with farmers. Tisquantum taught the pilgrims farming principles. Thus we know they had various agricultural skills.

Many societies have developed sustainable agricultural systems to produce crops for large populations. Before European contact, the Cherokee had produced and were farming at least 15 varieties of maize.

Spirituality has an impact on food production as well. The Three Sisters' crops for the Iroquis were maize, squash, and beans. We cultivate these three crops in our gardens in a complementary but advantageous grouping.

Spirituality has an impact on food production as well. The Three Sisters' crops for the Iroquis were maize, beans, and squash. We cultivate these three crops in our gardens in a complementary but advantageous grouping.

The Three Sisters have long represented young females' souls, collectively known as Our Life. Offerings and prayers of gratitude were made to these Three Sisters to express gratitude and appreciation for the crops.

This appreciation is an essential component of long-term viability. Most people in modern civilizations do not have it. The Wampanoag, a tribe who famously kept the Pilgrims alive in the first year, taught the Pilgrims numerous organic farming skills. They relied on nature for assistance.

Plants, like animals, need food, and the Wampanoag supplemented their diet with wood ash and fish scraps. These organic agricultural methods nurtured the land rather than depleted it.

Regenerative Agriculture (Permaculture)

Permaculture and regenerative agriculture are farming techniques that stress natural and holistic practices. Many Native Americans farm in the United States, with a substantial proportion being women. In truth, Native Americans/tribal nations own half of Arizona's agriculture.

The Hopi are well-known for their dryland agriculture. The southwest's arid atmosphere lends itself to this ancient method of farming. Hopi farmers today sow seeds deeper than was previously taught, and they utilize relatively little irrigation.

Ramona Farms, one of Arizona's largest Native-owned farms, is owned by the Button Family_ of Akimel O'odham (River People, Pima) of the Indian Gila River Community (commercial). In addition to commercial crops like alfalfa and cotton, they revived some old heritage plants formerly produced by southwest tribes.

They are cultivating the ball, a tepary bean that thrives in drought conditions. This is another example of working with your environment, land, and cultural legacy.

Foraging

Plant gathering in the wild is a wonderful way to reconnect with nature while augmenting our food source. When we quest wild foods, we may appreciate everything nature offers and the labor that goes into generating food for all group members.

Indigenous peoples taught us that foraging does not deplete the crop. We only harvest roughly one-third of a crop, leaving the rest to grow and reproduce. This ensures that there will be plenty for future generations and the next foraging expedition.

Foraging was also prized as a talent by Native Americans and early American colonists. It not only supplied food and flavoring ingredients but also medication. According to Iroquis archives, over eighty wild foods were obtained.

Hunting And Fishing

Fishing and hunting were common ways to add protein to one's diet. It was vital to use all of the animal parts that had been harvested. Throwing anything away was not an option.

Harvest celebrations were widespread among Native American tribes, celebrating food production and hunting.

Three deer were killed by local hunters. The rack and haunches were cut off, and the rest of the animal was left to rot. The waste and callous contempt for something as innocent as a white-tailed deer that had given their lives astounded me.

Religion And Spirituality

Native Americans have learned to coexist with nature rather than oppose it. This was mirrored in their culture. Native American faiths claimed they were spiritually connected to their natural Creator (s).

As we learned from the Iroquois Confederacy, Native Americans have recognized that their actions on the Earth impact future generations. Their forebears relied entirely on the land's resources, and we must respect that relationship.

They, like their forebears, wish to provide a stable future for their children.

Chapter 3: The Fundamental Values Of Native American People

Native Americans have a rich and diverse culture, one that is steeped in tradition. What might seem like a simple custom to you might be very important to them—or at the very least, they take it seriously. In this section, we're going to take a look at some of the foundational values of Native American people and see how they can help you create an effective marketing campaign. From concepts such as reciprocity and respect to imagination and intuition, these values will surely influence your marketing positively.

Integrity And Honesty

Native American people have long held strong values of integrity and honesty. These values are important because they help us stay true to ourselves and maintain our relationships with others.

Integrity means living up to our commitments, whether we make them to others or ourselves. Honesty is always telling the truth, even when it might hurt someone's feelings. We believe being honest is the best way to get along with others and keep our relationships healthy.

These values are important because they help us stay true to ourselves and maintain our relationships with others. They also help us work hard in everything we do. Suppose we can be honest with ourselves and others. In that case, we can focus on our goals without worrying about how people will judge us.

Prioritizing The Value Of Work Over Money

Money is not the most important thing in life. Work is. Native Americans have always placed a high value on work, which is why they are so successful as a people. Here are five fundamental values that Native Americans believe in and that guide their actions:

1) Respect: Native Americans respect others and their property. They don't take advantage of others and never abuse their power or authority. They know that if everyone respects each other, everyone will be able to live in harmony.

2) Responsibility: Native Americans take responsibility for their own actions and for the consequences of those actions. They know that good deeds will have positive results, and bad deeds will have negative consequences.

3) Cooperation: Native Americans cooperate with one another to achieve common goals. They know that working together is more effective than working alone, and it's more fun too!

4) Self-reliance: Native Americans rely on themselves rather than others for help or support. If something needs to be done, they figure out a way to do it themselves without outside assistance.

5) Fortitude: Native Americans are resilient, determined people who never give up on their goals, no matter how difficult the challenge may seem at first glance.

Appreciate The Role Of Women In Their Society

There is no one answer to the question of how fundamental women's roles in Native American society are. However, there are a few things that can be said with certainty. First, Native American women have played a vital role in shaping and sustaining the culture for centuries. Second, it is important to remember that Native American women have often been marginalized and even oppressed by men and society, which has led to them working harder than many other groups to maintain their cultural heritage. Third, it is necessary to appreciate the unique perspective that Native American women offer when considering the issues facing their people today.

Strong Bond Between Family Members And Society

Native American families have a strong bond with their society and its values. The family is the foundation of Native American culture and plays an important role in society. Families are responsible for raising their children, teaching them about their culture and traditions, and instilling in them the values that are important to them.

Family members are also responsible for upholding the cultural values of their tribe. They participate in ceremonies and rituals and contribute money and labor to support the community. Many tribes have chiefs or elders responsible for upholding the tribe's customs and traditions.

Native American families value relationships with other families. They often socialize together, sharing stories and recipes. They also help each other when needed, such as when one family member is sick or needs assistance with a difficult task.

Mutual Respect Towards One Another

Native Americans have mutual respect for one another and view themselves as part of the same community. This respect is based not only on shared traditions and values but also on kinship ties. Native Americans believe that all members of their community are responsible for upholding the culture and values of their tribe.

Tribal elders play an important role in fostering mutual respect among Native Americans. Elders are respected for their knowledge and experience and are often considered sources of wisdom and guidance. When conflicts arise, elders help to resolve them peacefully and democratically.

Native American people see themselves as stewards of the land and its resources. They take care not to damage or deplete natural resources and work together to protect sacred sites from development. In communities across the country, there are ceremonies honoring the Earth's spirit beings, who are seen as vital participants in preserving the environment.

Native Americans believe that it is important to live in harmony with nature. This philosophy has led many tribes to develop practices such as ecological agriculture, wildcrafting (using natural materials to create arts and crafts), eco-tourism, solar energy generation, and recycling programs.

Abide By The Natural Rules of Nature

There are a few things that Native Americans abide by that have been passed down from generation to generation. These natural rules of nature include honoring the land, the animals, and the spirits.

Honoring The Land

From the time we are born, we are taught to respect our land. We are not allowed to damage it or take what doesn't belong to us. Native Americans believe that everything on this earth is connected, and breaking these laws can negatively affect our ancestors and us.

The animals also play a big part in Native American culture. We see them as representatives of the Earth itself, and we treat them with the same respect we would want to be shown to us. We respect their space, their food sources, and their safety.

Spirituality And Religion

Native Americans believe in a spiritual world that is interconnected with ours. We call this world " Wakan Tanka," which means "Great Spirit." Every living thing has its own spirit; through ceremony and prayer, we can connect with these spirits and learn from them. This connection is important because it helps us understand our place in the world and how we can best care for our land and each other.

Respect Mother Earth

Ancient Native Americans considered Mother Earth alive, with a spirit and voice. They revered her as the provider of all life and the physical embodiment of everything sacred.

The principle guiding Native American respect for Mother Earth is tapu: a concept that encompasses our spiritual connection to the natural world and our responsibility to protect it. Tapu can be broken down into four main concepts: karakia (prayer), waiata (songs), manuhiri (landforms), and power (bodies of water).

Karakia refers to our acknowledgment of the Creator through prayer. We must always remember that we are one with everything, including Mother Earth, to keep her safe. Waiata is our music and oral history, which helps us connect with the spirits of nature. Manuhiri is what we call place names, landmarks, and other physical representations of our culture and heritage. PouWERi refers to bodies of water such as rivers, oceans, and lakes – where we gather for prayer, ceremony, and Hunt/Gather activities.

Generosity

There are many different and varied foundations upon which the Native American people have built their culture and society. These values range from generosity to respect for the land, all of which play a vital role in their lives.

One of the most important foundations upon which the Native American people have based their society is generosity. From sharing food with those who are hungry to lending a helping hand when someone is in need, the Native American people have always been generous. This generosity is not limited to interactions between individuals but extends to the community. For example, when a natural disaster such as a flood or hurricane, communities come together to provide aid and support to each other.

Another important foundation upon which the Native American people have based their society is respect for the land. From protecting sacred sites to taking care of the environment, the Native American people place great importance on respecting and taking care of the land. This respect helps ensure they can continue living in this country long after others have left it

Chapter 4: Herbalism History

Herbalism is one of the oldest and most essential fields of medicine. It has been used to treat various health problems for thousands of years. In this section post, we will take a detailed look into the history of herbalism and its role in modern medicine. We will explore the benefits and dangers of herbalism and the ingredients that make it such an effective treatment method.

What Is Herbalism?

Herbalism is the use of plants as medicines and remedies. Plants have been used for medicinal purposes for thousands of years, and many different types of herbal remedies exist. Herbalism is a complex topic, and there is still much to learn about it.

One type of herbal remedy that is often used today is dietary supplements. Dietary supplements are products meant to provide health benefits by supplementing the diet with ingredients traditionally claimed to be beneficial for human health. There are many different types of dietary supplements, including vitamins, minerals, herbs, and antioxidants.

There is evidence that some traditional herbal remedies may be helpful for certain diseases. However, there is currently not enough scientific evidence to support traditional herbal remedies as treatments for major diseases like cancer or Alzheimer's.

Where Did Herbalism Start?

Herbalism is one of the oldest sciences on earth. It dated back to the time before written language and was used by ancient people to heal themselves. Herbalism started with plants, and over time it has grown to include other aspects of natural medicine, such as Ayurveda.

Herbalism began with plants and is still primarily focused on plants today. However, over time herbalism has grown to include other aspects of natural medicine, such as Ayurveda. Ayurveda is a type of traditional Indian medicine that focuses on using herbs and other natural remedies to treat patients.

Herbalism During The Stone Age

Herbs to treat physical and emotional ailments date back to antiquity. During the stone age, people relied on herbalism to treat various health problems.

Herbalists during the stone age relied on plants for medication. They would identify the plant's characteristics and use them to cure specific ailments. These plants included angelica, dandelion, elderberry, lavender, nettle, rosemary, sage, and verbena.

Stone age herbalists would also use plant extracts to heal wounds. They would mix the extract with hot water and pour it over the wound. The herb would help draw out any infection and reduce inflammation.

Herbalism In Ancient Times

Herbalism has been around for centuries, and many different herbs have been used for various purposes. Some most common herbs include wildcrafted plants, tinctures, tea, and remedies. Herbalism can be used to treat a variety of health conditions, and it is also used as an alternative form of medication.

Herbalism has a long history with humans and humanoid species; herbaceous plants have been around for 125 million years. Thus the first humanoid beings did not appear until approximately 5 million years ago. All people were hunter-gatherers until about 12,000 years ago; this would be the longest period of human civilization. It's a lengthy and fruitful clinical trial aimed at discovering plants' medicinal and other potent properties.

Plants that provided the best food, weapons and fuels, medicines, colors, poisons, textiles, and hallucinogenic/spiritual encounters arose throughout this period. They all impacted people's minds, bodies, and society. The emergence of agriculture (approximately 10,000 years ago) and the establishment of more permanent communities in subsequent human history paved the way for a much more scientific approach to herbal remedies. Herbal medicine has been practiced for over 5,000 years, with only a few shards of information on preliterate herbal treatments.

According to archaeological evidence, medicinal plant use dates back to the Paleolithic epoch, some 60,000 years ago.

A guy was buried near Shanidar, Iraq, on a flower bed with plants such as Grape Hyacinth, Marshmallow, Henbane, Thistle, Yarrow, Ephedra, and others.

Studies of Neanderthal tooth plaques have also revealed that Neanderthals ate poplar, yarrow, and chamomile plants. The discovery of Otzi, a 5,300-year-old iceman from the Later Neolithic-Early Period, demonstrates ancient herbal expertise. He was discovered freezing and virtually hairless, with a backpack containing food, tools, and medicinal plants.

Otzi was carrying dried Sloe Berries from European Blackthorn, which appear to be a metabolic stimulant, immunological booster, carminative, anti-microbial, high in Vitamin C, anti-inflammatory, and anti-inflammatory Birch Polypore, a fungus having antiviral, vermifuge, and antibacterial characteristics. Both are considered cures for Whipworm, a parasitic nematode, and Lyme disease. The Sloe Berries had already been dried out from the previous fall, indicating that they had been employed for a specific purpose, hence Otzi's empirical knowledge of their medical properties.

Modern Day Herbalism

The history of herbalism spans back to before recorded history. The ancient Egyptians were some of the earliest documented practitioners of herbalism, using plants for healing purposes. Chinese herbalists developed a medical treatment system based on herbs more than 2,500 years ago. During the Middle Ages, herbalism was used to treat various illnesses. In modern times, herbalism has continued to be used for medicinal and recreational purposes.

Native American Herbalism

Native American herbalism is a centuries-old tradition that continues to be practiced today. Indigenous peoples across North America utilized plants for medicinal purposes. Their knowledge of these plants was passed down from generation to generation.

Some of the most common herbs used by Native Americans include sage, cedar, calamus root, dandelion, chicory root, wild mint, and Black Cohosh. These herbs were used to treat many issues, including headaches, colds and flu symptoms, toothaches, and pain relief.

Many tribes also used herbal remedies to promote fertility and increase energy levels. Herbal remedies were also used to prevent disease and heal wounds. Today, many Native Americans continue to use herbal medicine to treat a variety of health concerns.

Chapter 5: Herbalism And Modern Medicine

Native Americans carefully selected herbs that would benefit their communities and could use without endangering their health. Many medicinal plants were employed by indigenous peoples for healing. Some herbs and roots, for example, were crushed or eaten before being given to wounds as a first-aid therapy procedure. Others were boiled into herbal decoctions to cure fevers and diseases caused by bacteria; these therapeutic mixtures might also be coupled with other anti-microbial herbs or deadly plants.

It wasn't simply plants utilized for medicine; animals and minerals were also used to treat common ailments. Many people would treat rashes, wounds, or other skin ailments with a geode containing various cinnabar types (mercury sulfide). They would also ingest various stones as pills or liquids to excite their stomachs and aid in expelling intestinal gases. Several documented stories of rocks and other mineral medicine used for their healing powers throughout history.

A significant amount of effort was expended in identifying the most beneficial plants to the community, especially since many could cause harm if not used correctly. Many local plants were processed into a fine powder or decoction for medical purposes. To treat certain illnesses, including fever, gastrointestinal issues, and parasites, its powder or decoction would be mixed with water and drank. The plant's root bark, leaves, or seeds were used to make most of the decoctions; some species also utilized stones. The medications could be prepared from a single plant or a combination of several. Alcohol was occasionally added to each plant's therapy to make it flow more smoothly when taken.

Herbs were employed in ceremonies and daily life to prevent illness and maintain health. For example, the ancient curriculum of the Blackfeet tribe instilled in its kids the information and abilities required to become a skilled hunters. The young children were taught how to forage and prepare various medicinal herbs. They also learned how to harvest, clean, and process food plants. Herbs were utilized regularly to maintain health and prevent sickness.

Those looking for native plants must be respectful of the area and aware of the species they pick. Many of these locations are now protected by federal law because they have vital cultural importance for Native Americans. The American Indian Religious Freedom Act and the Endangered Species Act safeguard native plants. For example, the Native Grasslands

Protection Act was passed by Congress and protects endangered grasslands in six Western states, including Idaho and Montana.

It is crucial to note that many of these plants, particularly those found in high-altitude areas of Oregon and California, can only be found beneath rocks or cliffs. These areas are rich in wild medicinal plants, which can be easily overlooked if not searched since they are hidden within a rock fissure or have fallen over the cliff. Because of the loose dirt and rocky terrain, it is easy to become lost in these perilous areas. It is not advised to collect wild herbs in certain places.

The Native American relationship with medical herbs is prevalent today, with many of their natural treatments still in use. Native Americans have learned how to use natural resources in the wild to treat and preserve health. This expertise and tradition have been passed down from generation to generation with no reported loss of therapeutic understanding. We may preserve Native Americans' medicinal methods by teaching others how they used the herbs.

Picking is the contemporary term for gathering herbs, and the art of gathering herbs has numerous old names, including "gathering," "gatherin'," "picking," and even just plain "pickin'."

Every culture has its own traditional food preparation methods and medicinal herbs. Native American culture is one example.

Native American Herbal Medicine's Advantages and Applications

Herbal medicine is the use of plants to treat and even prevent a variety of disorders. As we all know, many ancient Native American societies used herbal medicine to maintain their health. Despite the advancement of contemporary science, more than half of the globe utilizes herbal therapy because it works.

- Affordability: Modern medicine has improved humanity's overall health so quickly, yet things are becoming more expensive, and accessing medical care is more complicated and difficult for many people than it is for others, and many people cannot afford things at this time.
- On the other hand, herbal medication is just as effective as modern treatment and costs far less. Another advantage of herbal medicine is that it works properly without adverse effects.
- Available in various forms: many people find it difficult to take any kind of medicine, whether herbal or pharmaceutical, and many people who cannot take it in one form will take it in another. Herbal medications can be purchased in various herbal shops, pharmacies, and even on the internet, allowing you to get your medicine in the most convenient manner. We recommend that consumers always ensure they get their herbs from a reputable source.
- Treatment efficacy: many herbal medications have undergone multiple trials, which have helped confirm the efficiency of these herbal medicines and ensure that they are safe for usage.
- Immunological-boosting properties: Herbal medicine helps to strengthen immune functions without interfering with the body's psychological processes; rather, it supports the body and aids in the maintenance of those processes. Everybody's component is increased to the point where it suddenly feels lighter and can function at its maximum potential.
- Native America is one of the birthplaces of herbal medicine, and their connection to nature was strong enough to recognize the benefits of specific plant treatments. This relationship has been translated to many parts of the world today, making it useful for many people.

Book 2: Native American Herbal Remedies

Chapter 1: Historical Overview Of Herbalism

Herbalism has a vast and varied history. It's practically hard to trace all of the significant herbalists who paved the path on one timeline!

While capturing centuries of herbal background in one place is difficult, a concise historical chronology provides a simple but essential picture of how contemporary herbalism came to be.

- 2800BC- The 'Pen Ts ao' is Shen Nung's first recorded herbal medication.
- c400BC- Happiness, nutrition, and exercise were all created by Hippocrates. It was composed in Greece around the year 1000 BC.
- c100BC - The first Greek herbal with illustrations appeared in.
- c50AD - Herbal medication and plant trade developed across the Roman Empire.
- c200AD - Galen, an herbalist, developed a system for classifying ailments and their respective treatments.
- c500AD- Myddfai's doctors followed Hippocrates' teachings. C800AD- Every monastery had an infirmary and a physic garden where monks experimented with natural remedies.
- c800AD- The Canon of Medicines was compiled by Avicenna, a physician. Throughout history, medicine and healing have been heavily influenced by Arab culture.
- 1200sAD- Herbalists successfully stopped the plague, not apothecaries who used arsenic and mercury and bled, purified, and prescribed it.
- 1500sAD- His Holiness Henry VIII advocated using herbal remedies. Medical practices have been regulated by several Acts of Parliament, including protection for "simple herbalists."
- 1600sAD- Herbs are available to the poor, but 'drugs,' derived from exotic plants, animals, or minerals, are reserved for the wealthy. Nicholas Culpeper authored 'The English Physician,' a classic herbal, in which he simplified the description of herbal medical practice.
- 1800sAD- Mineral-based pharmacological therapies began to encroach on herbal remedies. Over-the-counter versions of potent narcotics like laudanum and mercury were widely accessible, and reports of their harmful consequences began to surface. Herbal medicine has fallen out of favor due to the explosive growth of the pharmaceutical business and now seems 'outdated.'
- 1900sAD- The invention of penicillin and the rise of the pharmaceutical industry after World War I led to a dramatic increase in global pharmaceutical production. There are still just a few herbalists practicing this ancient art. The Pharmacy and Medications Act of 1941 revoked the powers of herbalists to prescribe medicines to patients. The Act has never been implemented because of public outrage.
- 2000AD- Currently, European law mandates that all herbal medications be tested in the same manner as conventional pharmaceuticals. All-natural treatments would, after that, be permitted on the market. Meanwhile, the UK government assesses the likely consequences and people's opinions of this law.

Chapter 2: Common Diseases Treatable With Herbs

think of herbs, they think of traditional remedies like peppermint tea for headaches or lavender oil for relaxation. But there's a whole world of herbs out there that can be used to treat diseases and illnesses. This section will explore some of the most common herbs used to fight disease and illness. By learning about these herbs and their properties, you can better identify which ones might be useful for treating your health issues.

Abdominal Pain

There are a variety of causes for abdominal pain. The most common is indigestion, or GERD, caused by the overproduction of stomach acids. Other causes include gallstones, ulcers, and tumors. Many diseases and illnesses can be treated with herbs, including:

-Indigestion: Try gargling with salt water or taking an over-the-counter anti-indigestion medication such as Pepcid AC (famotidine) or Prilosec OTC (omeprazole). If these don't work, try using a tablespoon of ginger mixed with a cup of warm water before meals.

-GERD: Treating GERD means avoiding acid reflux, which can be done by altering your diet and lifestyle factors, such as avoiding drinking alcohol and eating smaller meals multiple times a day instead of one large meal. You may need to take medications to relieve your symptoms if all else fails.

-Gallstones: Take fiber supplements like psyllium husk powder (Metamucil) or choline bitartrate (Centrum). A stone can sometimes be removed surgically.

-Ulcers: Ulcers are often caused by allergies or infections that reach the gastrointestinal tract. Treatment typically includes antibiotics and analgesics to reduce inflammation and pain, along with surgery if necessary.

-Tumors: More than 80 percent of malignant tumors originate in the GI tract

Aches

Many diseases and illnesses can be treated with herbs. Here is a list of some of the most common: headaches, sore throats, colds, flu, bronchitis, and asthma. Herbs can also treat other conditions, such as digestive problems, menstrual cramps, and skin issues.

ADHD

Attention-deficit hyperactivity disorder (ADHD) is a mental health condition characterized by problems with focus, hyperactivity, and impulsiveness. While there is no single cause for ADHD, it is believed to be caused by a combination of genetic and environmental factors. Symptoms usually develop in children between 6 and 12 but can persist into adulthood. There is currently no cure for ADHD, but treatments include medication, counseling, and behavior modification therapies. Herbal remedies can also help treat ADHD symptoms, as many herbs have anti-hyperactivity properties.

1. Ginkgo biloba extract: Ginkgo biloba is an extract from the ginkgo tree that has been used traditionally in China to treat Alzheimer's disease and other cognitive issues. Researchers believe ginkgo Biloba may also be effective in treating ADHD because it has anti-hyperactivity properties. One study found that ginkgo Biloba helped reduce impulsivity and increase focus in people with ADHD.

2. Passionflower extract is another herb commonly used to treat anxiety disorders and other conditions. Some studies have suggested that passionflower may also effectively treat ADHD symptoms such as impulsiveness and hyperactivity. In one study, participants who took passionflower extract experienced significant improvements in their attention span and distractibility compared to placebo recipients.

Alzheimer's Disease

Alzheimer's Disease is a progressive neurodegenerative disorder that affects memory and thinking. There is no cure currently available, but herbal remedies are being studied as possible treatments.

One study found that the herb ginkgo Biloba can improve memory in Alzheimer's patients. Ginkgo contains compounds that may protect the brain from damage caused by the disease. Another study found that the herb rosemary can reduce symptoms of Alzheimer's in mice. Rosemary is known to help improve cognitive function and memory in humans.

Other herbs studied for their potential effects on Alzheimer's include Co-enzyme Q10, omega-3 fatty acids, and chamomile tea.

Anemia

Anemia is a deficiency of hemoglobin in the blood. This can be caused by several problems, including iron deficiency, disease, and medications. Several herbs can help treat anemia.

Herbs traditionally used to treat anemia include berberine, ephedrine, garlic, ginger, licorice, and vitamin C. Some newer options include red yeast rice and black cohosh.

Speaking with a healthcare provider about which herbs might be best for you is important. Also, discuss any other symptoms you are experiencing related to your anemia.

Anxiety

There are many different types of anxiety; each person experiences it differently. Some people experience a generalized anxiety disorder characterized by persistent and excessive worrying about numerous things. Other people have panic disorder, characterized by recurrent attacks of intense fear that can last for minutes or hours. Still, other people have a social anxiety disorder, which is the fear of being embarrassed or judged by others.

Treating anxiety with herbs is very effective in many cases. Here are some of the most common herbs used to treat anxiety: valerian (Valeriana officinalis), hops (Humulus lupulus), kava (Piper methysticum), lavender (Lavandula angustifolia), lemon balm (Melissa officinalis), chamomile (Matricaria chamomilla), passionflower (Passiflora incarnata) and St. John's wort (Hypericum perforatum).

Appendicitis

Appendicitis is a serious medical condition that can lead to death if not treated quickly. Appendicitis is caused by appendages - small, movable parts of the large intestine - becoming blocked, usually due to infection. The appendix can become inflamed (red and hot) and surrounded by fluid.

Without treatment, appendicitis can lead to peritonitis (a serious injury to the inner lining of the abdominal cavity), which can lead to death. Treatment for appendicitis typically includes surgery to remove the appendix. Herbal treatments have been used for centuries to treat various illnesses and injuries, and many herbs effectively treat appendicitis. These herbs include dandelion root, burdock root, goldenseal root, mistletoe berries, chickweed, red clover flowers, horsetail tea, white willow bark extract, and opium poppy oil. Suppose you are experiencing signs or symptoms of appendicitis. In that case, it is important to seek professional medical help as soon as possible.

Bed Wetting

Several diseases and illnesses can be treated using herbs. Bedwetting is one such condition.

Bedwetting is a medical condition in which a person experiences excessive urination at night. This can be caused by various reasons, including stress, anxiety, or a nervous disposition.

If left untreated, bed wetting can lead to problems such as bladder infections, urinary tract problems, and even kidney stones. Herbs can help treat bedwetting by helping to reduce the stress and anxiety that may be causing the problem. Additionally, herbs can help relieve bedwetting symptoms such as bladder pain or discomfort.

Bloating

Many diseases and illnesses can be treated using herbs. Some of the most common ones include:

1. Acid reflux disease: One of the most common causes of stomach pain is acid reflux, which can be treated with herbs such as ginger or peppermint.

2. Bronchitis: A cold or the flu can cause bronchitis, a respiratory infection that usually affects the lungs. Over-the-counter cough medicines and herbal remedies such as echinacea can help to treat bronchitis.

3. Constipation: Many people experience constipation at some point in their lives, and several effective herbs can help to remedy the problem, including ginger, dandelion, and fennel.

4. Cystic acne: This type of acne is caused by an overproduction of sebum (a natural oil). Herbs such as rosemary, thyme, and sage are excellent treatments for cystic acne because they contain compounds that block sebum production.

Broken Bones

In the world of herbs, there are many ways to heal broken bones. Herbs can be used both topically and internally. Topical application is when the herb is applied to the injury site. This method is most effective immediately after the bone has been broken. Herbs can be used internally before or after a bone has been fractured. There are a variety of herbs that have been proven to aid in healing bone fractures and other injuries. Below are some of the most commonly used herbs for this purpose:

Turmeric is one of the most popular herbs for healing bone fractures (Curcuma longa). Turmeric is a yellow spice that comes from India and Pakistan. It has been used as an herbal remedy for centuries and is often recommended for its anti-inflammatory properties. When applied topically, turmeric has been shown to help speed up the healing process and reduce inflammation. Additionally, it has been shown to promote new cell growth and increase the strength of connective tissue

Another popular herb for healing bone fractures is garlic (Allium sativum). Garlic was first mentioned in ancient Greek writings as a medicinal plant that could help heal wounds and improve health overall。 Garlic is one of the oldest medicines known to man. It has been used throughout history as a natural treatment for various illnesses。 Garlic extract can be applied topically to help speed up the healing process while maintaining beneficial anti-inflammatory properties 。

Boils

There are many boils, but a pustular boil is the most common. Pustular boils are caused by bacteria that grow rapidly in warm, moist areas. This type of boil is often found on the face or neck.

The first step in treating a pustular boil is to identify the cause. If you know that it's caused by the Staphylococcus aureus bacteria, you can reduce the bacteria in your environment and treat the boil with antibiotics. If you don't know what caused it, your doctor will likely prescribe an antibiotic based on the type and location of the boil.

Once you've identified and treated the cause, you'll need to keep an eye on the boil for signs that its healing. Boils can rupture and spread infection if not treated quickly. So always seek medical attention if you have a pustular boil and see any signs of infection such as redness, drainage, or pus.

Bruises

Bruises can occur from various sources, such as falls or being hit with an object. They can be very painful and may take a long time to heal. There are many types of bruises, and the best way to treat them depends on the cause.

If the bruise is caused by falling, it is important to immobilize the area with a bandage or splint. If the injury was from being hit with something, it is important to get medical help immediately. Bruises vary in size and color, but they all need treatment to heal properly.

Burns

Burns is one of the most common injuries in the United States, with over 600,000 cases treated in hospitals each year. There are many different burn types, each requiring a unique treatment plan. Here is a list of some of the most common types of burns and their corresponding treatments:

First-degree burns are the least serious type of burn and require no treatment other than cool water applied to the burn area several times a day.

Second-degree burns involve partial loss of skin tissue and require first aid measures such as cooling the burned area with cold water or ice, applying pressure to reduce swelling, and removing any dirt, debris, or clothing that may be covering the burn.

Third-degree burns involve total loss of skin tissue and necessitate medical attention, including intravenous fluid therapy and antibiotics to prevent infection. Many third-degree burns also result in permanent scarring.

Fourth-degree burns involve deep gashes or open wounds that may require surgical intervention to close them. These types of burns are very serious and can lead to extensive damage.

Common Cold

The common cold is a viral respiratory infection that can be treated using herbs. Herbal remedies are safe and effective; many people find them more comfortable than traditional treatments. The most common herbs to treat the cold include echinacea, garlic, goldenseal, and ginger.

Constipation

Constipation is a common problem that can be treated with herbs. Many herbs relieve constipation, including ginger, dandelion root, and licorice. These herbs stimulate the digestive system to help waste matter pass through the body more easily. Other herbs that help relieve constipation include lavender, fennel, and catnip. Some people relieve constipation by taking a natural laxative such as buchu or senna.

Dementia

Dementia is a condition that results in significant memory loss and difficulty performing complex tasks. Many causes of dementia, including Alzheimer's disease, are the most common form. Other causes include stroke, brain tumor, and head trauma. While there is no cure for dementia, many treatments are available to help patients live better lives.

One type of treatment for dementia is cognitive rehabilitation therapy. This therapy helps patients learn new skills and improve their overall functioning. Another type of treatment is medication therapy. Many medications are available to treat dementia; each may have different benefits and drawbacks. It is important to discuss any potential treatments with a doctor before starting them.

Cognitive rehabilitation therapy can be very helpful for people with dementia. It teaches them new skills, such as cooking or cleaning, which can help them live more independently and reduce caregiver stress. Occupational therapies can also be used alongside cognitive rehabilitation therapy to help people with dementia continue working or pursuing other activities they enjoy.

While there is no cure for dementia, many treatments are available to help patients live better lives. Cognitive rehabilitation therapy is one such treatment that has shown promising results in reducing symptoms and improving function overall.

Diarrhea

Diarrhea is a common problem, and there are many ways to treat it. One of the simplest ways to treat diarrhea is to drink plenty of water and eat salty foods to make the body less thirsty. Some people also recommend taking over-the-counter diarrhea remedies like Bisacodone or Pepto-Bismol. If these remedies don't work, your doctor may prescribe a specific antibiotic or antidiarrheal medication. You can also try easing the symptoms with herbal remedies. Some popular herbs for treating diarrhea include aloe vera gel, ginger, hops, peppermint oil, and turmeric. Consult with your doctor before using any herb as a treatment for diarrhea, as some may not be safe for pregnant women or children.

Hair Loss

Hair loss is a common problem, and there are many treatments available. There are various causes of hair loss, including genetics, stress, and illness. Treatment options include medications, surgery, hair restoration, and natural remedies.

Migraine

Migraine is a dreaded disorder that affects over 30 million people in the United States. It is a type of headache that typically occurs on one side of the head, lasting from four to 72 hours. Unlike other types of headaches, migraines are characterized by their pulsating quality and their tendency to occur with light or noise exposure.

Migraine is caused by a combination of genetic and environmental factors. Research has found that women are more likely to experience migraines than men, and they tend to occur during certain phases of the menstrual cycle. However, no single cause has been identified for all cases of migraine.

There is currently no cure for migraines, but many treatments available can help relieve symptoms. Some common remedies include over-the-counter painkillers such as ibuprofen or naproxen, prescription medications such as triptans (such as Excedrin Migraine) or ergotamines (such as Elavil), and natural therapies such as ginger or turmeric. Some lifestyle changes may also be necessary, such as avoiding stressful situations or drinking alcohol excessively.

Herpes

Many diseases and illnesses can be treated using herbs. Herpes, for example, is a virus that can be treated with herbal remedies. Herbal remedies work by attacking the root cause of the infection rather than just treating the symptoms. Many herbal remedies can help treat herpes, and it is important to find one that will work best for you. Some of the most common herbal remedies to treat herpes include ginger, garlic, and cayenne pepper.

Impotence

If you're experiencing erectile dysfunction (ED), many traditional and alternative remedies are available. One alternative treatment is herbalism. Several herbs have been traditionally used to treat ED, some of which are quite potent. Here are three herbs that can help improve your libido:

Gentian is a herb that has been traditionally used to boost libido. It works by increasing blood flow to the genitals, which can improve sexual arousal and performance.

L-arginine is another herb that is effective in treating ED. It helps with blood flow and increases penile rigidity.

Finally, Rhodiola Rosea is a popular herb for improving overall energy levels and boosting the immune system. It's also been shown to help treat ED.

Kidney Stones

Kidney stones are a common problem, affecting up to 10 percent of the population. They can form when the urine becomes too concentrated, and small stones form. Stones can also form from an obstruction in the urinary tract, such as a stone in the bladder or kidney. Stones can become lodged in the kidney, leading to pain and difficulty urinating. There is no cure for kidney stones, but many treatments can help relieve symptoms.

Many people find relief from kidney stones by drinking plenty of fluids and eating a high-fiber diet. Some people also use natural remedies, such as kidney stone pills or supplements. These remedies may include oxalate-fighting herbs like turmeric or dandelion root, diuretics like cranberry juice or iced tea, and minerals like potassium citrate. Surgery may be necessary to remove a stone blocking the flow of urine or filter out smaller stones that cannot be removed through other means.

Malaria

Malaria is a dangerous and potentially deadly infection caused by the protozoan parasites Plasmodium falciparum and P. vivax. The parasite enters your body through the mouth, nose, or skin and can cause fever, chills, sweating, muscle pain, and fatigue. Malaria can lead to seizures, coma, and even death in severe cases. There is no cure for malaria, but treatments include medications to reduce fever and inflammation, antimalarial drugs to kill the parasites inside your body, and mosquito netting to keep them out. Some herbs have been proven to help protect against malaria infection in preliminary studies; however, more research is needed before these herbal remedies can be recommended as standard treatments for this disease.

Menstrual Cramps

The menstrual cramps that many women experiences are often treatable with herbs. Many herbs used to treat menstrual cramps also treat other types of pain, such as arthritis and migraines. Common herbs used to treat menstrual cramps include ginger, borage oil, chamomile, lavender oil, and peppermint oil.

Morning Sickness

Morning sickness is a common condition that affects up to 20% of pregnant women. Morning sickness may be mild, moderate, or severe and can last from a few days to more than a week. There is no one cause of morning sickness. Still, it may be caused by environmental changes (like travel), food (especially bland foods), hormones, infections, or stress.

There is no specific cure for morning sickness, but many treatments available can help relieve symptoms. Some treatments include over-the-counter medications (such as ibuprofen or acetaminophen) or prescription medications (such as domperidone or ondansetron). Other treatments include dietary changes (like eating bland foods), drinking lots of fluids, resting, and acupuncture. If symptoms are severe, hospitalization may be necessary.

Nausea

Nausea is a common symptom associated with a variety of diseases and illnesses. While several treatments are available, many can be effective in conjunction with other treatments. Some of the most commonly treated causes of nausea include gastroenteritis, cancer, pregnancy, and morning sickness.

There are many types of herbs that can be used to treat nausea. Herbs such as ginger, lavender, mint, and ginger root can help reduce nausea symptoms. Other herbs, such as turmeric and licorice, can help reduce inflammation or vomiting. Many herbal remedies can be found at health food stores or online. When choosing an herbal remedy to treat nausea, you must speak with a healthcare professional about the best option.

Book 3:
Native American Herbalism Encyclopedia Vol 1

Chapter 1: The Bases Of Native American Herbalism

Like many other Native American tribes, Cherokee medicine was passed down through generations to "selected" healers. Traditional Cherokees sought medical experts' advice on various issues, from medical concerns to personal conflicts and emotional difficulties. Similar cures for colds, aches and other minor ailments were used by other Native American cultures.

The Circle Of Medicine

Coughs, sore throats, and diarrhea were commonly treated with boneset tea and wild cherry bark among Cherokee and other Native American tribes. A tea produced from the roots of Blue Cohosh was traditionally used to alleviate childbirth discomfort and hasten delivery. Diabetes patients may benefit from Devil's Club and Wild Carrot Blossoms. Teas made from Feverwort, Dogwood, and Willow bark were found to help relieve common cold symptoms.

In the past, wild lettuce, wild black cherry, and hops were all used to create sedatives for big procedures. Penicillin, for example, began as a Native American cure before making its way into modern medicine.

The Circle of Medicine

2000 BC - Take a bite out of this root.

1000 AD - That is a heathen root. Say this prayer here.

1500 AD - That prayer is based on folklore. Take this potion and drink it.

1940 AD - Snake oil is the name of the potion. Take this tablet and consume it.

1985 AD - That medicine isn't working. Take this antibiotic from here.

2007 AD - That antibiotic is no longer effective. Take this root and devour it!

Medicine Wheel and 4 Directions of Native Americans

Native Americans have a strong connection to nature, which they use to create and maintain balance, health, and well-being. "Mother Earth" is referred to, and her significance has been incorporated into various ceremonies and traditions. One example is the medicine wheel, which metaphorically represents both completion and the circle of life.

The Medicine Wheel comes in a variety of shapes and sizes. It could be an item, a painting, or a concrete structure on the ground. Indigenous peoples in North America have erected dozens of Medicines Wheels over the years.

The Medicine Wheel and Native American ceremonies follow a round pattern, often clockwise or "sun wise." This makes synchronizing easier with natural forces such as gravity and the sun's rising and setting.

The Meaning Of The Four Directions

Various cultures interpret the Medicine Wheel differently. For others, each of the four directions (East, West, North, South) is represented by a different color, such as black, white, red, and yellow, which signifies the human race. The Directions could also point to anything in the image below:

Direction	Stages of Life	Season	Elements	Animal	Plant	Heavenly Body	Colour
North	Elders & Death	Winter	Wind	Bear	Cedar	Stars	White
East	Birth & Children	Spring	Fire	Eagle	Tobacco	Sun	Yellow
South	Youth	Summer	Water	Wolf	Sweetgrass	Earth	Black
West	Adults & Parents	Autumn	Earth	Buffalo	Sage	Moon	Red

Chapter 2: The Best 200 Medical Herbs To Use

Agave

Agaves are a type of succulent plant native to the United States. There are over 100 different species of agaves, ranging in size from small plants that can be tucked away in a corner to large specimens that can reach 10 feet tall. Agaves are used for their succulent leaves, flowers, and fruit. Some benefits of using agaves include reducing stress, improving blood circulation, fighting inflammation, and providing antioxidants.

Alder

The alder tree is common in many parts of the United States. Native to North America, the alder is a hardy tree that can grow in dry and moist environments. The bark of the alder is rough and scaly, and the leaves are alternate, with serrated margins. The flowers are small and green, and the fruit is an acorn. The male and female trees produce different types of acorns.

The sap from the alder tree can be used to make syrup, beer, vinegar, soap, glue, paper, plastics, dyes, and other products. The wood from the alder is also useful for furniture making, construction materials, and other items. The bark can also be used as an astringent or to treat cold and flu symptoms. The roots of the alder plant contain chemicals that can be toxic if consumed in large quantities. However, the roots can also be used to treat various medical conditions.

Alder

There are over 1,500 different types of native American herbs. Many of these herbs have been used for centuries by indigenous people for various purposes, such as healing, promotion of fertility, and protection from pests and disease.

Some of the most popular native American herbs include:

Alder (Alnus rubra) is a common tree in many parts of North America. The bark is used to make a tea believed to help treat colds and other respiratory ailments. The leaves and branches also make remedies for digestive problems, arthritis, skin conditions, and more. Alder wood has been historically used to build furniture and tools. The flowers are used to make wine and honey.

Aloe Vera

Aloe Vera is a succulent plant that originates from Africa. It can grow up to four feet tall and have fleshy, green leaves with white stripes. The plant produces yellow flowers, which are pollinated by bees. Aloe Vera has been used for medicinal purposes for centuries and is now also being studied for its possible health benefits.

Some potential benefits of aloe Vera include reducing inflammation, providing relief from pain and swelling, and improving skin health. It is also an effective natural detoxifier and has antimicrobial properties. Some people use aloe Vera as a treatment for acne, varicose veins, psoriasis, eczema, and other skin conditions.

Amaranth

Amaranth is an ancient, gluten-free grain that packs much nutritional punch. It's a great source of fiber, vitamins, minerals, and antioxidants. Here are some of the benefits of eating amaranth:

1. It's high in fiber: One cup of cooked amaranth has 10 grams of fiber, which is more than any other grain! This can help to keep you feeling full longer and help promote regularity.
2. It's packed with vitamins and minerals: Amaranth is a good source of vitamin B6 (an important nutrient for red blood cells) and Vitamin C (which helps to fight off infection). It also contains copper, magnesium, potassium, and phosphorus.
3. It's a healthy weight loss option: Amaranth is low in calories and has a low glycemic index, meaning it won't cause spikes in your blood sugar levels after meals. This makes it a great choice if you want to lose or maintain your current weight.
4. It has antioxidant properties: Amaranth is high in antioxidants, including lutein and zeaxanthin – two types of carotenoids linked with cancer prevention.

Amaranth

Amaranth is an ancient grain known for its health benefits. This grass-like plant can be found growing wild across North America. Here are three of the most notable benefits amaranth can provide:

1. Amaranth is a great source of iron, essential for healthy and red blood cells.
2. Amaranth is also a good source of vitamin B6, which helps to keep your brain and nervous system running smoothly.
3. Amaranth is a good source of fiber, which can help to promote better digestion and reduce the risk of obesity and heart disease.

American Licorice

Native American licorice is a plant that can be found throughout North America. This plant treats various health problems, including respiratory issues and diarrhea. Licorice is also known to improve heart health and boost energy levels.

Some other benefits of licorice include reducing inflammation, promoting joint health, and decreasing anxiety and stress. It is also believed to have anti-cancer properties.

American Mistletoe

The American mistletoe (Viscum album) is a hardy, fast-growing vine that can reach heights of 10 feet or more. The plant has white flowers and edible red berries. The root and leaves have medicinal properties, including effective against colds, coughs, and injuries. The mistletoe is also used in herbal remedies to treat anxiety, low blood pressure, bronchitis, and other conditions.

Angelica

Many native American herbs have been used for centuries to treat various ailments. Some of the most well-known and popular include angelica, ginger root, lavender, and garlic.

Angelica is a herb with many benefits for health. For example, angelica is purported to help improve heart health by reducing inflammation and helping clean the blood. Additionally, angelica is effective in treating hypertension and other cardiovascular conditions. Additionally, angelica can help improve digestion by promoting healthy bacteria colonies in the gut.

Ginger is another herb that has numerous benefits for health. Ginger is known to be an effective pain reliever and can also help reduce inflammation. Additionally, ginger can help improve circulation and joint function and stimulate the immune system. In addition to its health benefits, ginger is also delicious!

Antelope Sage

The antelope sage, Salvia pratensis, is a perennial bush that grows 2 to 4 feet in height. The leaves are oppositely arranged, and the branches are stout. The flowers are bell-shaped and blue or purple in color.

The antelope sage has many benefits, including helping to reduce inflammation, relieve pain, promote healing, and calm anxiety and stress. It is also an anti-inflammatory agent to treat respiratory issues such as bronchitis and asthma.

Arnica

Arnica is a flower that is native to the Alps. Arnica contains various compounds, including arnica Montana lactone, which has anti-inflammatory and analgesic properties. Arnica also has vasoconstrictor properties and can be used topically to treat wounds and other skin injuries.

Ashwagandha

ashwagandha (Withania somnifera), also known as Indian ginseng, is a plant native to India and Nepal. It has been used as a traditional herbal medicine in the region for centuries. Ashwagandha has been studied for its potential to improve cognitive function, reduce anxiety and stress, and improve sleep quality.

Aspen

This hardy tree grows quickly to 12-20 feet tall, has narrow leaves and produces fragrant white or pink flowers in late spring. The bark is rough and reddish-brown, with small, knotty needles. The sap is used to treat wounds and other skin problems and is made into throat lozenges. Wood is also used to make furniture, tools, and arrows.

Astragalus

Astragalus is a genus of flowering plants in the legume family, Fabaceae. There are about 20 species, all native to North America. Many of the species are used by Native American tribes as part of traditional medicine.

Some of the species in the genus are used medicinally as supplements or as ingredients in traditional remedies. Astragalus membranaceus is known especially for improving blood flow and reducing inflammation. Astragalus sinicus, another species in the genus, has been traditionally used for treating heart disease and other conditions affecting the cardiovascular system. The roots and stems of some species in the genus are also edible and may be used to make tea or food dishes.

Attractylodes

Attractylodes is a genus of about 20 flowering plants in the lily family. They are native to North America and grow in moist areas such as stream banks and seeps. Many of the species are used by Native Americans for medicinal purposes. Some species are used to treat colds, sore throats, respiratory infections, and stomachaches. Some species' leaves and stems are also eaten raw or cooked.

Balsam Fir

Balsam Fir is a native North American tree that can grow up to 40 feet tall. It has triangular leaves and fragrant, cone-shaped flowers. The sap from the balsam fir can be used to make balsam oil, which is used for treating skin conditions and as a fragrance agent. The balsam fir tree is also known for its medicinal properties, including the treatment of inflammation, pain relief, and respiratory problems.

Balsam Root

Balsamroot is a perennial herb typically growing to a height of 1-2 feet. The leaves are lance-shaped and have serrated edges. The flowers are small, green, and borne in clusters at the top of the stem. The root contains copal resin, which treats skin conditions and promotes healing. Balsamroot has been used for centuries by Native Americans as an herbal remedy for a variety of ailments. It is also known for its anti-inflammatory properties, which make it beneficial for treating arthritis and other forms of pain. In addition, balsam root is an effective treatment for reducing stress and anxiety.

Barberry

Barberry (Berberis aquifolium) is a member of the barberry family native to North America. These shrubs typically grow up to 3 feet tall with spiny branches and small leaves. The flowers are bell-shaped and white, and the fruit is a purple drupe. The shrub has been used by Native Americans for medicinal purposes for centuries.

Some benefits of using barberry include improving circulation, reducing inflammation, healing wounds, and promoting detoxification. This herb's antiviral and antibacterial properties make it a valuable addition to any health regimen.

Bearberry

Many amazing native American herbs have a wide range of benefits, from treating minor illnesses to aiding in overall wellness. Here are five of the best bearberry plants for your medicinal garden:

Blue Cohosh (Campsis radicans)

This herb has been traditionally used to treat menopausal symptoms such as hot flashes and vaginal dryness. It also helps improve blood flow and menstrual cramps.

Bearberry (Arctostaphylos uva-ursi)

One of the most popular bearberries, black bearberry is an excellent choice for those looking for an anti-inflammatory and antioxidant plant. It can be useful for treating skin conditions like eczema and managing other menopausal symptoms like hot flashes and vaginal dryness.

Bee Pollen

Bee pollen is one of the most popular natural supplements on the market. Native Americans have been using bee pollen for centuries to improve their health and wellness. Bee pollen is a high-quality source of protein, fiber, vitamins, minerals, and antioxidants. Some benefits of bee pollen include improved immune system function, better sleep quality, and reduced inflammation.

Beech

Beech is a hardy tree that can grow in a variety of environments. Beech trees are good for beekeeping, providing nesting sites and food for honeybees. The leaves and twigs of the beech tree are used to make beer, wine, and spirits. The wood of the beech tree is also used to make furniture, cabinets, and other items.

Beeswax

Beeswax is a natural wax made by honey bees. It can be used as a cosmetic or furniture polish. Beeswax is also used in some pharmaceutical products.

Black Chokecherry

Black chokecherry (Prunus serotina) is a small, deciduous tree that grows up to 25 feet tall. The fruit is a dark purple cherry, and the bark is smooth with dark flecks. The leaves are ovate, the margin crenate (serrated), and the flowers are white with pink petals.

The black chokecherry is native to the eastern United States and can be found in low-lying areas near water. It prefers moist, acidic soil and can grow in full sun or shade. The tree is drought-tolerant but does best when watered regularly during active growth periods.

Black chokecherry is noted for its medicinal properties, which include anti-inflammatory properties, antiviral properties, and antioxidant properties. It has been used historically to treat conditions such as rheumatoid arthritis, gout, and fever. The tree is also used as a food source by wildlife species such as deer and turkey.

Black Cohosh

Black Cohosh is a North American herb used for centuries to treat various health conditions. The plant is typically found in moist areas near bodies of water. It has been traditionally used as a female contraceptive to relieve menopausal symptoms. Additionally, black Cohosh treats hot flashes, anxiety and depression, sexual dysfunction, and menstrual cramps. Some Common Uses for Black Cohosh

1) Female Contraceptive: Black Cohosh is traditionally used as a female contraceptive because the plant contains compounds that can prevent ovulation.

2) Menopause Relief: Black Cohosh is also popularly used to relieve menopausal symptoms such as hot flashes, night sweats, mood swings, and fatigue. In studies, black Cohosh was more effective than other traditional treatments such as hormone replacement therapy (HRT) or antidepressants.

3) Anxiety & Depression: Several studies have shown that black Cohosh can help reduce anxiety and depression symptoms in people who struggle with those conditions.

4) Hot Flash Relief: Black Cohosh has also relieved hot flash symptoms.

Black Gum

Ephedra is a popular black gum native American herb that has been used for centuries as a stimulant and treatment for asthma and other respiratory issues. Cranberry root is known for purifying the blood and removing toxins from the body. In contrast, the dandelion root is a natural anti-inflammatory agent. Garlic and ginger are both well-known spices that have medicinal properties. At the same time, yarrow is an effective herb for treating pain, anxiety, depression, and menstrual cramps.

Black Haw

Black haw is an essential herb for Native Americans. It has been used for centuries to treat various ailments. The plant is also known for its antibacterial and antiviral properties, making it a valuable addition to any healthcare regimen. Here are five benefits of using black haw:

1. It helps to fight infection.
2. It alleviates inflammation.
3. It can help improve circulation.
4. It can reduce pain and swelling.
5. It has anti-inflammatory and antioxidant properties, which can fight against aging and promote health overall

Black Raspberry

The Black raspberry is a hardy shrub that can grow up to 4 feet tall and 2 feet wide. The leaves are ovate-shaped, and the flowers are magenta. The fruit is black when ripe and contains two seeds. The Black raspberry has medicinal properties and is used to treat various ailments such as arthritis, bronchitis, colds, gastritis, heartburn, headache, indigestion, kidney stones, muscle aches, or toothache. Additionally, the leaves can be brewed as tea to treat ailments such as insomnia or stress.

Bloodroot

Bloodroot is a wildflower that grows in the eastern and central United States. The root treats various health problems, including skin infections, digestive issues, and pain. Bloodroot is also used to improve memory and cognitive function.

Bloodroot

Bloodroot is a perennial herb that can be found throughout North America. This herb has been used by Native Americans for centuries to treat a variety of medical conditions. Bloodroot contains anti-inflammatory and antioxidant compounds, making it a popular choice for treating pain and inflammation. Some benefits of bloodroot include reducing inflammation in the joints, reducing stress levels, and improving mood swings.

Blue Cohosh

Blue cohosh is a perennial herb that grows up to one foot high. The leaves are ovate, lance-shaped, and blue-green in color. The flowers are small, white, and purple. The root is fleshy and fibrous. Blue cohosh has been used as a traditional medicine by Native Americans for centuries. It is believed to have properties that help improve sexual function, relieve pain, and increase circulation. Some benefits of using blue Cohosh include improved moods, fertility, and relief from menstrual cramps.

Blue False Indigo

Blue False Indigo is a type of wildflower native to North America. This herb has been used by Native Americans for centuries for medicinal purposes. Blue False Indigo has a variety of benefits that can be used by people today.

Blue False Indigo is known to help improve circulation and reduce inflammation. It can also treat colds, flu, and other respiratory infections. Additionally, false blue indigo can help improve the complexion and reduce wrinkles.

Blue Spruce

This herb treats many health problems, including inflammation, colds and flu, and asthma. It boosts the immune system and can help relieve headaches and tension headaches. It can also reduce anxiety and depression symptoms.

Blueberry

Native American herbs have many benefits that can be enjoyed by people of all ages. They are high in anti-inflammatory properties, which can help ease chronic pain and arthritis symptoms. Some of the best blueberry herbs include elderberry, Oregon grape, and wild berry.

Each of these plants has specific benefits for your health. Elderberry is a natural anti-inflammatory that can help reduce pain from arthritis and back pain. Oregon grape is a potent source of antioxidants, which can protect your cells from damage and may improve your overall health. Wildberry is an excellent source of vitamins, minerals, and anthocyanins, all of which support good health.

Boneset

Boneset (Eupatorium perfoliatum) is a perennial herb found in moist areas of the eastern United States. The root and leaves are used medicinally, the root being the most commonly used part. Boneset has been used to treat chest pain, anxiety, bronchitis, and other respiratory ailments for centuries. The stems, root bark, leaves, and flowers are all considered to have medicinal properties.

Some benefits of a boneset include reducing inflammation and fever, promoting a healthy immune system, and aiding digestion. Additionally, it has been known to help reduce stress and improve moods. Some reports also show that bonesets can effectively treat epilepsy and other neurological conditions.

Boswellia

Boswellia is a genus of about 40 trees and shrubs in the pea family Fabaceae. The plants are endemic to the hot, dry deserts and semi-arid areas of North Africa, the Middle East, India, and Australia. The active ingredients in Boswellia oil (Boswellia serrata) are responsible for its therapeutic effects.

The oil is extracted from the fruit or resin of Boswellia serrata trees by cold pressing. It contains up to 80% alpha-boswellic acid, which has anti-inflammatory properties. In traditional medicine, Boswellia oil is used to treat many problems, including pain relief from arthritis and other medical conditions; inflammation; skin problems such as eczema and psoriasis; and problems with breathing such as asthma. Some studies have also shown that it can help improve cholesterol levels and protect against heart disease.

Broom Snakeweed

Broom snakeweed (Glechoma hederacea) is a perennial herb that grows to around 1 meter in height. It has smooth, somewhat wiry leaves and produces small, delicate flowers. The plant is native to the eastern US and grows in moist areas such as bogs, swamps, and stream banks.

The root of broom snakeweed contains several glycosides used by Native Americans for centuries for medicinal purposes. These include berberine, barbaloin, squalenone and squalane. Some of these glycosides have anti-inflammatory properties and can be used to treat conditions such as arthritis, asthma, and Crohn's disease.

Other benefits of broom snakeweed include improving blood circulation and reducing inflammation caused by injuries or diseases. The plant is also a natural source of antioxidants which can help protect the body from damage caused by free radicals.

Buck Brush

Buckbrush is a native perennial herb found in the Rocky Mountain region of North America. The plant is often used to help promote relaxation and relieve stress. It has been traditionally used as a natural remedy for headaches, anxiety, and depression. Buckbrush also has antibacterial and antifungal properties that can help treat infection.

Buckthorn

Buckthorn (Rhamnus cathartica) is a shrub or small tree that can grow up to 6 feet tall. The leaves are opposite, elliptical, and measure 2 to 4 inches long and 1 inch wide. The flowers are reddish-purple, and the fruit is a dry capsule.

The bark is smooth, scaly, and reddish-brown. The twigs are covered with soft hairs. The fruit is a tart berry that contains oxalic acid (a compound that can irritate the skin).

The leaves and bark of buckthorn have been used for medicinal purposes for centuries. Buckthorn was used by Native Americans to treat wounds, inflammation, colds and flu, diarrhea, indigestion, stomachache, and other ailments. Some of the benefits of using buckthorn include: reducing pain, and fever reduction, stopping bleeding, helping improve circulation, boosting the immune system, fighting infection, and treating skin problems such as psoriasis.

Buffalo Berry

Buffalo Berry (Elymus canadensis)

The Buffalo Berry is a perennial herb found throughout much of North America. The roots and stems are used to make medicine, and the leaves and flowers are edible. The Buffalo Berry has been used for hundreds of years to treat various ailments, including diabetes, cancer, heart problems, respiratory issues, and more. Here are some of the benefits of using buffalo berries:

1. It helps control blood sugar levels
2. It helps reduce inflammation
3. It can help improve heart health
4. It can help improve respiratory health
5. It is an antioxidant and can fight against free radical damage

Burdock

Burdock is a herbaceous plant found in many different parts of North America. It has been used for centuries by Native Americans for medicinal purposes. Burdock is packed with nutrients and has many health benefits. Here are five of the best:

1. Burdock is a good source of both dietary fiber and antioxidants. According to a study in the "Journal of Medicinal Food," burdock extract had antioxidant activity comparable to some well-known antioxidants such as vitamin E and resveratrol. This helps protect cells from damage caused by free radicals, which can contribute to various diseases such as cancer.

2. Burdock is also high in calcium. One cup (120 grams) of cooked burdock contains 176 milligrams of calcium, which is more than twice one cup (60 grams) of milk! That's because burdock contains significant amounts of oxalic acid and phytate, which bind up minerals like calcium, so they cannot be absorbed by the body. However, boiling or steaming the burdock before eating will break down these inhibitors, allowing more calcium to be absorbed into your bloodstream.

3. Burdock is a good source of vitamins A and C. One cup (120 grams) of cooked burdock contains 16 percent DV (daily value) of vitamin A and 5 percent DV of vitamin C, both important nutrients

Calamus Root

Native American herbs have long been used by tribal healers to promote health and well-being. Calamus root is one such herb, revered for its healing properties. Here are some of the benefits of using calamus root:

1. Calamus Root Can Help Relieve Anxiety and Stress Levels

Calamus root is effective in relieving anxiety and stress levels. This is partly due to its ability to stabilize moods and alleviate symptoms such as irritability, restlessness, insomnia, and tension headaches.

2. Calamus Root Can Aid in Detoxification

One of the main benefits of using calamus root is its ability to aid in detoxification. It enhances the body's natural eliminative processes, including the kidneys, liver, intestines, lungs, and skin. This can help clear out unhealthy toxins from the body and promote overall health and well-being.

3. Calamus Root Can Help Improve Digestion

Another benefit of using calamus root is its ability to improve digestion. It helps break down food so it can be absorbed into the bloodstream more easily, promoting overall digestive health and well-being.

California Poppy

California poppy (Eschscholzia californica) is a native North American herb used medicinally for centuries. It is an antioxidant, anti-inflammatory, and anti-anxiety agent. California poppy also helps to reduce stress and anxiety, improve sleep quality, and boost mood.

There are many benefits to using California poppy as a natural remedy for stress and anxiety. It relieves restlessness, fatigue, insomnia, irritability, tension headaches, muscle pain and stiffness, shakiness, and dizziness. Additionally, California poppy can help boost mood and relieve depression or sadness.

Cardinal Flower

The cardinal flower (Lobelia cardinalis) is a perennial herb that grows in central and eastern North America. The flowers are pink, white, or purple and are typically 1-1.5 inches wide. The root system of the cardinal flower is extensive and can be used for medicinal purposes. Some benefits of using the cardinal flower include treating colds, flu symptoms, headaches, anxiety, and menstrual cramps.

Cascara Sagrada

Cascara sagrada is a rare and potent compound found in the bark of the Pacific yew tree. The herb has been used for centuries by Native Americans as a natural treatment for various health problems, including seizures, high blood pressure, and joint pain.

Cascara sagrada has been shown to have numerous benefits regarding overall health. For example, studies have shown that the compound can help lower blood pressure and slow the growth of cancer cells. Additionally, cascara sagrada has improved cognitive function and reduced anxiety and stress symptoms.

The best way to take cascara sagrada is by consuming the extract or tincture form. Be sure to speak with your doctor before beginning any herbal therapy. All supplements should be taken cautiously and under their guidance.

Cat's Claw

Cat's Claw (Uncaria tomentosa) – also known as Indian hemp, badger brush, and yerba santa – is a plant that grows in the United States and parts of Canada. It has long been used by Native Americans for medicinal purposes, and scientists believe it may have health benefits. Cat's claw contains compounds that may help reduce inflammation and pain, improve blood circulation, and protect the heart. Some people also use it to treat arthritis and other conditions.

Catnip

The plant "Catnip" has long been used as a remedy for numerous ailments. It is thought to have sedative, antispasmodic, and analgesic properties. Recent studies have shown that catnip can also be beneficial to the heart.

Cattail

A cattail is a plant found in many lakes and rivers. This plant grows from one to two feet high and has long slender stems. The leaves are medium green and have an oval shape. The flowers are small and white. Cattail is a good source of fiber, vitamins A and C, potassium, magnesium, and calcium.

Cayenne

Cayenne is a hot pepper plant native to South America. The Cayenne pepper is used in many types of cuisine, such as Mexican and French cooking. It has a moderate heat level, so it is a good choice for those who want some heat but don't want to be overwhelmed. Cayenne peppers are also great for adding flavor to food without overpowering it.

Some of the benefits of using cayenne peppers include the following:

-They can help reduce inflammation and pain due to arthritis and other conditions

-They are good for relieving symptoms of colds and flu, such as congestion and fever

-They can improve circulation and help boost the immune system

Cedar

Cedar is a member of the Pine family and grows in many different parts of the world. Wood from cedar is used for many things, including building materials, furniture, and sculptures. Cedar oil has many uses, including treating skin conditions and hair care products.

Chamomile

Chamomile is a flowering plant that grows in many parts of the world. It has been used for centuries as a medicinal herb and is now known to have a host of health benefits. Chamomile effectively reduces anxiety and stress, improves sleep quality, and relieves pain. It also possesses anti-inflammatory properties, which can help to reduce the symptoms of conditions like arthritis.

Chickweed

Chickweed (Stellaria media) is an important plant in Native American herbal medicine. Chickweed has been used as a treatment for various health issues for centuries and is still used today. Chickweed contains a variety of beneficial compounds that can help improve overall health.

One of the primary benefits of chickweed is its ability to reduce inflammation. Antioxidants found in chickweed have been shown to help protect the body from damage caused by free radicals, common inflammation causes. Chickweed is a powerful stimulant, and it has been used to treat conditions like fatigue and insomnia.

Chickweed also has antimicrobial properties that can help fight infection. In addition to killing harmful bacteria, chickweed may also inhibit the growth of other types of fungus. This makes it an effective treatment for chronic infections such as Lyme disease and Candida overgrowth.

Chlorella

Chlorella is a single-cell plant known to improve cognitive function and reduce inflammation. This microalgae can also help reduce the risk of heart disease, diabetes, and stroke.

Some of the potential benefits of chlorella include:

1) improved cognitive function
2) reduced inflammation
3) reduced risk of heart disease, diabetes, and stroke

Chokeberry

Chokeberry is a shrubby vine that typically grows up to 4 feet tall. It has fragrant pink or white flowers that are pollinated by bees. The fruit of the chokeberry is a dark red berry that can be eaten fresh or used in cooking.

There are several benefits to taking chokeberry supplements or eating its fruit. For example, chokeberry has been shown to improve heart health by reducing inflammation and promoting blood flow. It can also help prevent some forms of cancer by fighting tumors from forming and by boosting the immune system. Also, chokeberry may help improve cognitive function and memory recall in people suffering from Alzheimer's disease or dementia.

Cinnamon Bark

Cinnamon is a spice with a rich history and many uses. Cinnamon bark is the dried inner bark of a tree species in the laurel family. The bark is dark brown and has a strong, sweet smell.

Cloves

Cloves are a spice that comes from the underground stem of an evergreen tree native to Madagascar. Cloves are often used as a flavoring agent in foods and beverages. Still, they can also be used in natural medicine. Some benefits of clove include reducing inflammation and pain, improving mood and memory, and protecting the lungs.

Club Moss

Club Moss is a potent herb used by the Sioux and other North American tribes for centuries. The leaves and stems of this plant are used to make a tea or infusion that is thought to have various benefits. These include reducing inflammation, treating respiratory problems, and boosting the immune system.

Some of the specific benefits attributed to club moss include:

-Reducing inflammation: Using club moss as an herbal remedy may help reduce inflammation, improving conditions such as arthritis.

-Treating respiratory problems: Club moss may also be effective in treating respiratory issues such as bronchitis and asthma. This is because it contains compounds that help relax air passages and improve airflow.

-Boosting the immune system: Club moss may also help boost your immune system by increasing the production of white blood cells.

Coltsfoot

Coltsfoot (Aconitum napellus) is a member of the Ranunculaceae family and native to temperate Eurasia and North America. In addition to its traditional use as a pesticide, Coltsfoot was historically used for treating fever, gastrointestinal problems, and arthritis. The herb is also purported to treat anxiety and depression, enhance nervous system function, improve fertility, and protect the liver.

Corn

Corn is a versatile plant for various purposes, including food and fuel. Corn is a source of dietary fiber, carbohydrates, and other nutrients. The plant also contains antioxidant compounds and is a good source of protein. There are many health benefits associated with eating corn, including reducing the risk of heart disease, diabetes, and some types of cancer.

Cranberry

Cranberry is a small, shrubby, deciduous tree that can reach heights of 10-15 feet. It has smooth, thin bark and produces oval-shaped fruit that ranges in color from light green to deep red. The tart fruit is used in juice, sauce, jams, and cranberry jelly. The plant's leaves are arranged in pairs, and its flowers are pollinated by bees.

Creosote Bush

Creosote bush is a member of the Asteraceae family. The genus name, Creosote, is derived from the Greek word for resin. This plant is found in Central and Western North America.

The creosote bush grows to a height of 1-3 meters. It has opposite leaves that are ovate to oblong in shape, with entire margins and a serrated edge. The inflorescence contains up to 50 yellow flowers that may be bisexual or unisexual, with five petals reflexed at the base and fused at the tip. The fruit is a capsule that opens to release two shiny brown seeds.

The creosote bush is used as an herbal remedy for various conditions. It is thought to be effective in treating fever, inflammation, and respiratory problems. It has also been used to treat joint pain, skin diseases, nerve disorders, and digestive problems. Some studies have shown that it may help reduce the risk of cancer.

What are the benefits of using creosote bush?

The benefits of using creosote bush include:

-It is effective in treating fever

-It can help reduce the risk of cancer

-It has been used to treat joint pain, skin diseases, nerve disorders, and digestive problems

Damiana

Damiana (Damiandra Zizanoides) is a member of the mint family and grows wild in Mexico and Central America. The leaves and flowers of damiana are used to make tea, extract oil, and treat a long list of ailments. Damiana has been used for centuries by indigenous people in the area as a cure-all, but modern research has suggested its benefits.

The tea made from damiana is said to be a stimulant, diuretic, and aphrodisiac. It is also thought to help reduce anxiety, stress, and insomnia. Extracts from the plant have been found to help treat anxiety disorders, depression, nerve pain, menstrual cramps, fertility issues, skin conditions including psoriasis and eczema, memory problems, and more.

Damiana can also help improve circulation and reduce inflammation. In addition to these traditional uses, recent research has shown that damiana may also help improve cognitive function in older adults and promote healthy cell growth.

Dandelion

Dandelion is an excellent plant for detoxifying the body. It contains a high amount of vitamin C, making it great for fighting off sickness. Additionally, dandelion is packed with antioxidants that help to protect cells from damage. Other benefits of consuming dandelion include improved liver function and better digestion.

Devil's Club

In North America, the plant Devil's Club is most commonly found in the Coastal Mountain Range of California and Oregon. The plant is a member of the Buckthorn family and can grow up to 12 feet tall. Devil's Club has a long history of use as a medicinal plant, with traditional usage including treating ulcers, cancer, and infections. The plant contains secondary metabolites that have been shown to have health benefits, including anticancer properties.

Dogbane

Dogbane is a genus of plants in the sunflower family. The species are native to North America and include the common dogbane (Duguetia Versicolor), the dwarf dogbane (Duguetia minima), and the prickly dogbane (Aconitum napellus). Dogbane flowers are typically purple or blue and have five petals, each with a long filament. The root system is fibrous and parasitic.

The dogbane flowers are used as a tea for treating inflammation, fever, and other conditions. The plant is also used to calm nerve pain and treat insect bites. The root system contains azulene oil, which has anti-inflammatory properties. Additionally, the plant contains flavonoids and tannins that benefit skin health and hair growth.

Dogwood

Native American herbs are some of the most versatile and beneficial plants on the planet. These natural remedies can help improve your quality of life from healing wounds to boosting overall health. This section will look at ten of the best Native American herbs and their benefits.

Dong Quai

Dong Quai is a well-known Chinese herb used for centuries as a natural remedy for various health conditions. In particular, Dong Quai is commonly used to treat menopausal symptoms, anxiety, and stress. Some other benefits associated with Dong Quai include improved nerve function, better sleep quality, and relief from joint pain.

Some key compounds in Dong Quai include dong Quai oil, dong Quai root extract, and dong Quai bark extract. All three of these ingredients have been shown to have powerful anti-inflammatory properties. They have also been shown to improve blood flow and circulation, which helps reduce inflammation throughout the body.

There are many different ways to enjoy Dong Quai supplements. You can purchase them over the counter or in some health food stores. They are also available online. Suppose you're looking to take a Dong Quai supplement regularly. In that case, it's best to talk to your healthcare provider first since some potential side effects can be associated with taking this herb regularly.

Douglas Maple

Douglas Maple is a hardy, fast-growing tree in many parts of the world. It is a popular tree for landscaping and produces a high yield of sugar maple syrup. The tree is also known for its strong branches and ability to resist pests and diseases. Some health benefits associated with Douglas Maple include improved circulation, relief from joint pain, and reduced anxiety.

Eastern Skunk Cabbage

Eastern Skunk Cabbage (Portulaca oleracea) is a North American native plant that is often used as a culinary herb. The plant has a long history of use as an herbal remedy for various ailments and is often considered a powerful detoxifier. Eastern Skunk Cabbage can also treat or prevent gastrointestinal problems like indigestion and constipation. Additionally, the plant is said to be beneficial for overall brain health and function and skin health. Some other benefits associated with Eastern Skunk Cabbage include reducing inflammation and swelling, helping to promote healthy hair and nails, and improving digestion.

Echinacea

The plant "Echinacea" is native to North America and has been used as a medicinal plant for centuries. Echinacea is a member of the daisy family and is known for its ability to improve circulation and fight infection. Some of the health benefits of using Echinacea include relief from colds, flu, sinus infections, and other respiratory ailments and boosting the immune system.

Elderberry

Elderberry is a shrub that can grow up to 3 feet tall, with leathery leaves and clusters of small white or pink flowers. The berries are edible and have a sour taste. Elderberry is used in traditional medicine to treat colds, flu, and other respiratory ailments. The plant also has health benefits beyond the treatment of common illnesses. Elderberry has been shown to help reduce cholesterol levels, improve blood sugar control, and reduce the risk of heart disease.

Eleuthero

Eleuthero is a genus of flowering plants in the family Araliaceae. The generic name is derived from the Greek words eleutherios (ἐλευθερισμός, meaning free from fear) and this (τίκτος, meaning bush). There are about 30 species in the genus, most of which are endemic to Siberia and North America. Of these, only two – Eleutherococcus senticosus and Eleutherococcus palustris – are known to occur outside those regions.

Despite their limited distribution, indigenous people have long used eleuthero plants as medicine. They are particularly well-known for their benefits in treating anxiety and stress-related disorders and Russian colds and other respiratory infections. Some species have also been shown to improve immune function and reduce inflammation.

The most common constituents of eleuthero plants are terpenes, including sabinene, cineole, camphene, β-pinene, limonene, myrcene, and α-terpineol. These compounds exhibit a wide range of medicinal properties, including antioxidant activity, anti-inflammatory properties, and anticancer properties. In addition to their traditional medicinal uses, some terpenes have recently been identified as potential biofuel sources.

Eucalyptus

The eucalyptus tree is native to eastern Australia and New Caledonia. The tree grows up to 30 meters tall and has smooth bark that is red-brown in the older trees. The leaves are ovate and lanceolate, with a pointed apex and a serrated margin. The flowers are white or pink, with five fused petals at the base. The fruit is a capsule that splits open to release the seeds.

The eucalyptus tree has many benefits for Native Americans. One of the benefits is that the tree can be used as a natural pesticide. The leaves have antifungal properties and can be used to treat common lawn diseases such as downy mildew and rust. Another benefit of the eucalyptus tree is that it has anti-inflammatory properties. This means that it can be used to treat conditions such as arthritis and headaches. Additionally, the oil from the eucalyptus tree has been shown to have antiviral properties, meaning it can be used to treat colds and flu infections.

Evening Primrose

Evening primrose (Oenothera biennis) is a flowering plant that grows in temperate regions of the world. The plant has been used as a traditional medicine and has been shown to have several health benefits. These benefits include reducing inflammation, improving heart health, and helping to improve joint function.

Fendler's Bladderpod

The Fendler's bladderpod, also known as the bladderpod lily or the American bladderpod, is a perennial herb native to North America. It grows up to 1.5 feet tall and has oval-shaped leaves that are green on top and white on the bottom. The flowers are purple and have yellow centers.

The Fendler's bladderpod is used in herbal medicine for its anti-inflammatory properties, ability to soothe digestive issues, and ability to fight infection. It is also used for treating skin conditions, calming anxiety, and regulating blood sugar levels.

Fennel

If you're looking for a natural remedy for minor health concerns, look no further than the Fennel plant. Native Americans have used fennel since pre-historic times to treat health issues such as indigestion, diarrhea, and respiratory problems. The plant is also known to improve mood and cognitive function. Here are six reasons why you should add this herb to your regular diet:

1. Fennel fights against gas and bloating.
2. It helps improve digestion and relieve constipation.
3. It has anti-inflammatory properties that can help relieve pain and inflammation.
4. It has antioxidant properties that fight against harmful free radicals in the body.
5. It can help reduce anxiety and stress levels in the body.
6. Finally, fennel is a good source of dietary fiber, which can help regulate blood sugar levels and promote overall intestinal health

Fenugreek

Fenugreek (Trigonella foenum-graecum) is a flowering plant that belongs to the family Fabaceae. Fenugreek is native to India and Pakistan and parts of south-central Asia. Fenugreek is also cultivated in other parts of the world, including North Africa, the Middle East, and Europe. Fenugreek has been used medicinally for centuries in various parts of the world. The leaves and seeds are used for medicinal purposes.

Feverfew

Feverfew (Tanacetum parthenium) is a plant found in Europe and Asia. It is used as a traditional remedy for various health problems. The plant is thought to have anti-inflammatory, analgesic, and fever-reducing properties.

Feverwort

Feverwort is a popular native American herb that has many benefits. It is used to treat colds, flu, and other respiratory infections. Feverwort also has anti-inflammatory properties and can help relieve pain. It is also beneficial for the heart and circulatory system.

Galangal

Galangal is a rhizome that grows in Southeast Asia and is used as a spice. The extract from galangal is used in Asian cuisine to flavor dishes. Some of the benefits of using galangal include:

1. Galangal can help increase circulation and improve sleep quality.
2. It has anti-inflammatory properties, which can help reduce pain and inflammation associated with conditions such as arthritis and joint pain.
3. It can also help improve digestive function, especially when used with other herbs such as ginger and turmeric.

Garcinia Cambogia

Garcinia cambogia has become a popular weight-loss supplement in recent years. However, there is limited research on the effectiveness of this extract for weight loss. Some studies have shown that Garcinia cambogia can help you lose weight, while others have not. The National Center for Complementary and Integrative Health (NCCIH) has not evaluated the safety and efficacy of Garcinia Cambogia for weight loss.

Garlic

Garlic is one of the most popular plant herbs due to its many health benefits. It is high in allicin, which has antiviral properties and antioxidant properties that protect cells from damage. Garlic can also help reduce inflammation throughout the body and improve blood flow. In addition to these traditional uses, garlic is also effective at treating.

Gentiana

Gentiana is a genus of flowering plants in the sunflower family. The genus is native to North America and commonly found in dry or sandy habitats. There are about 20 species in the Gentiana genus, most of which are herbs. Some of the species in the Gentiana genus are used for medicinal purposes.

Some benefits of using gentian plants include acting as an appetite stimulant and helping reduce stress levels. Some gentian plants are also used for their cosmetic properties, helping to promote hair growth and preventing skin irritation.

Ginger Root

Ginger root is a versatile herb that has been used medicinally for centuries. The ginger root contains many compounds with therapeutic benefits, including anti-inflammatory and analgesic properties. It can be used to treat a variety of conditions, including headaches, stomach cramps, and fever. Ginger root also has antiviral and antibacterial properties, making it a useful tool in treating infections.

Ginkgo Biloba

Ginkgo biloba is a venerable tree found in many parts of the world. Still, it's especially well-known for its benefits to the human body. Native to China and Japan, ginkgo Biloba is a favorite herb of traditional Chinese medicine because it improves circulation, memory function, and stamina.

The ginkgo tree has also been used in Eastern Europe to treat diabetes and other diseases. It contains terpenes, flavonoids, and other antioxidants that help fight off disease. The ginkgo Biloba extract is an effective treatment for dementia and Alzheimer's. In addition to these individual benefits, studies have shown that regular use of ginkgo Biloba can help prevent age-related cognitive decline and keep people sharper mentally into their older years.

Ginseng

Ginseng is a plant that has been used for centuries to improve health. It has various benefits, including improved energy levels, reduced stress, and better mental clarity. Some of the health benefits of ginseng include decreased risk of cancer, better blood circulation, enhanced libido, and improved immune system function.

Glucomannan

Glucomannan is one of the most popular and beneficial native American herbs. Glucomannan is a type of fiber that helps regulate blood sugar levels, promotes weight loss, regulates cholesterol levels, and provides many other benefits.*

Glucomannan can be found in foods like seaweed, fruits, vegetables, and grains. However, it is best to supplement with it since most foods don't contain enough glucomannan. Adding glucomannan to your diet can help improve your overall health and well-being.*

Goldenrod

The goldenrod plant is a slow-growing perennial that is native to North America. The plant has been used medicinally for thousands of years and has been found to have various health benefits. These benefits include reducing inflammation, treating anxiety and depression, aiding in cognitive function, and helping to improve circulation.

Goldenseal

Goldenseal (Hydrastis Canadensis) is a plant used for centuries to treat various ailments. The plant contains berberine, which is known to have anti-inflammatory, antibacterial, and antiviral properties. It has also been effective in treating arthritis and other joint conditions. There are many health benefits to taking goldenseal supplements, including reducing the risk of cancer and helping to improve overall digestion.

Gooseberry

Gooseberry is a small shrub that grows up to 2 feet tall. It has leaves that are close to the ground and blue flowers that are pollinated by bees. Gooseberry is a type of berry that grows in temperate zones worldwide. The berries are eaten fresh, dried, or made into jams, jellies, syrups, and wine. Gooseberry has many health benefits because it contains vitamins C and K, fiber, and antioxidants.

Gravel Root

Gravel root is a plant native to North America. It has been used for centuries by Native Americans for medicinal purposes. It is now being studied for its health benefits, specifically for treating anxiety and depression.

In animal studies, gravel root has been shown to reduce anxiety and depression symptoms. It also increases GABA levels, a neurotransmitter that helps regulate mood. Additionally, gravel root has anti-inflammatory properties, which could help treat arthritis.

Green Hellebore

There are many types of native American herbs that have been used by Native Americans for centuries for their medicinal properties. Many of these herbs have been identified as effective in treating various ailments, including anxiety, arthritis, heart disease, and more.

One perennial herb particularly well-known for its medicinal properties is green hellebore. This plant has been used by Native Americans to treat a variety of conditions, including anxiety and depression. In addition to its traditional uses, green hellebore has also been found to help treat cancer and other diseases.

Some benefits of using green hellebore include reducing anxiety and depression symptoms, improving heart health, reducing inflammation, and preventing cancer. Green hellebore may be a good option for you if you are looking for an herbal remedy that can help improve your overall health.

Green Tea

There are many benefits to green tea, whether for general health or specific ailments. The antioxidants in green tea help protect the body against various diseases, while the catechins provide numerous health benefits.

Green tea can be consumed as a beverage, cooked into dishes, or used as a topical treatment. Drinking green tea consistently has reduced the risk of developing cancer and other chronic diseases. Additionally, green tea's ability to boost cognitive function has led to its use as a mild stimulant for improved concentration.

One downside of consuming large quantities of green tea is that it can cause nausea and an upset stomach. When purchasing green tea, read labels and select those made from organically grown leaves.

Guarana

Guarana (Piper guarana) is a shrubby tree that can grow up to 25 feet tall. The bark is rough, and the leaves are oppositely arranged with serrated margins. The flowers are white and small, and the fruit is a capsule. Guarana is native to South America and is found in Brazil, Paraguay, and Uruguay. It has been used by the indigenous people of these countries for centuries as a stimulant and anti-inflammatory agent.

The native people of Brazil chew the leaves to get their desired effects. The caffeine in guarana beans has been historically used to treat problems such as headaches, fatigue, anxiety, depression, and insomnia. Guarana also helps promote better mental clarity and focus before or after physical activity. Some people also use guarana to increase energy levels during workouts or other vigorous activities.

Gymnema Sylvestre

Gymnema Sylvestre is a botanical indigenous to North America commonly found in the eastern and central United States. The plant is used for various purposes, such as memory enhancement, anxiety relief, and improving circulation.

The herb has been used for centuries by Native Americans as a means of enhancing memory, reducing anxiety, and treating cardiovascular disease. Modern-day trials have shown that Gymnema can improve circulation and restore cognitive function in patients with Alzheimer's disease or other forms of dementia.

Hawthorne

Hawthorne is a plant that has been used for centuries for its medicinal properties. It is known for improving mental clarity, reducing anxiety and depression, and helping to promote a healthy immune system. Additionally, Hawthorne is a natural source of antioxidants, which can help reduce the risk of cancer and other diseases.

Book 4:
Native American Herbalism Encyclopedia Vol 2

Chapter 1: The Best 200 Medical Herbs To Use

Heal-All

Heal All is a plant that has been used for centuries by indigenous tribes all over the world to heal wounds and ailments. The plant is both antibacterial and antifungal and is effective in treating various skin conditions, such as eczema, psoriasis, and dermatitis. Additionally, Heal All is beneficial in treating infections such as colds and flu and respiratory problems such as bronchitis.

Hibiscus

Native American herbs are often used for medicinal purposes. Some of the most popular and well-known Native American herbs include hibiscus, dandelion, and rose hips. Hibiscus is a flowering plant that is native to North America. The flowers are purple with a yellow center and are used for juice, tea, or perfume. Dandelion is also native to North America and is known for its medicinal properties. The flowers can be eaten fresh or dried and have been used to treat various ills, from hair loss to congestion. Rose hips are also native to North America and are high in antioxidants and vitamins C and A. They are used in herbal teas, tonics, salad dressings, baked goods, etc.

Honeysuckle

Honeysuckle (Lonicera japonica) is a flowering plant that belongs to the Caprifoliaceae family. It is native to China, Japan, Korea, and Russia but is also cultivated in many other parts of the world. The plant grows as a shrub or small tree and can reach heights of up to 10 feet. The flowers are white or pink and are produced in clusters at the ends of branches.

Hops

Hop is a flowering plant in the family Humulus lupulus. It is a climbing plant that grows up to 2 meters tall. The hop plant produces a bitterness-sweet flavor in beer and other alcoholic beverages. The flowers are pollinated by bees, and the hop bines make hops products, such as malt.

Horse Gentian

When it comes to finding out about the best native American herbs, you have several options at your disposal. One such herb is horse gentian. This plant has a long history of use by Native Americans and has been known to help with various issues. Here are some of the benefits that can be attained from using horse gentian:

- boosts energy levels
- helps to improve cognitive function
- supports cardiovascular health
- promotes healthy skin and hair growth
- reduces inflammation and pain

Horsetail

The horsetail plant is a perennial herbaceous plant that can grow up to 2 meters in length. It has a long, thin stem that can become woody at the base and strap-like leaves. The horsetail plant contains over 200 compounds, including essential oils, that have been used for centuries for medicinal purposes. Some of these compounds have been shown to have health benefits, such as anti-inflammatory and antiviral properties.

Indian Ginseng

Indian ginseng is a popular herbal remedy used in Asia for centuries. The root of this plant is used to treat several health conditions, including fatigue, depression, and memory loss. Indian ginseng is also known to improve circulation and energy levels.

Some benefits of using Indian ginseng include increased focus and concentration, better sleep quality, and reduced anxiety and stress. It is also thought to help reduce inflammation and promote overall well-being.

Indian Hemp

Indian hemp has been used to treat anxiety, depression, and other mental health disorders. It has also been used to improve sleep quality and reduce the occurrence of nightmares. Indian hemp is also effective in treating other medical conditions, such as chronic pain, inflammation, and seizures.

Some of the most common uses for Indian hemp include:

-Treating anxiety and depression

-Improving sleep quality

-Reducing the occurrence of nightmares

Indian Paintbrush

The Indian Paintbrush is a flowering plant in the daisy family. It grows 3 to 4 feet tall and has narrow leaves and small white or pink flowers. The root system is strong, and the plant can survive in dry or moist environments. People have been using Indian Paintbrushes for generations for their medicinal properties.

Indian Paintbrush treats various ailments, including pain, inflammation, and fever. The flowers also help treat anxiety, depression, memory loss, and other cognitive problems. Some people even use Indian paintbrushes as insect repellent.

Indian Paintbrush is native to North America and can be found throughout the eastern United States, Canada, and Mexico.

Ironwood

Ironwood is a type of tree that is native to North America. Wood from ironwood is highly prized for its strong, durable qualities. The tree is also known for its medicinal properties, which include being effective against infections and providing relief from pain. Ironwood has several health benefits, including reducing inflammation, fighting cancer, and improving heart health.

Jame's Buckwheat

Jame's buckwheat, also known as Eriogonum jamesii, is a wildflower in the western United States and Canadian provinces of British Columbia and Alberta. Jame's buckwheat is a herbaceous perennial plant that grows to 1 foot in height. The leaves are ovate-elliptic in shape and have smooth edges. The flowers are pink or white and are located at the top of the stems. The fruit is a capsule that contains one or two seeds.

Jame's buckwheat has numerous benefits for both human health and the environment. For human health, the plant contains high levels of antioxidants which can help protect cells from damage caused by toxins and free radicals. Additionally, the plant has anti-inflammatory properties, which can help reduce inflammation-associated diseases such as arthritis. For the environment, Jame's buckwheat helps to improve soil quality by providing nutrients needed for plant growth and helping to bind particles together so they can be more easily removed by rain or snow runoff.

Jiaogulan

Jiaogulan, or Gynostemma pentaphyllum, is a traditional Chinese herb that improves circulation and energy levels. It has long been recognized as a powerful antioxidant with healing properties for the skin and other organs. In recent years, scientists have also discovered that jiaogulan may help reduce stress and anxiety, improve sleep quality, boosting cognitive function, and reducing inflammation.

The most common use of jiaogulan is as a dietary supplement to improve general health and well-being. Jiaogulan can be taken as a tea, tincture, capsule, or extract. There are many different ways to take jiaogulan, so find the method that works best for you. Some people prefer to take it in the morning before breakfast, while others take it in the afternoon or at night before bed.

Some benefits of taking jiaogulan include improved circulation, better sleep quality, reduced stress, and anxiety symptoms, increased cognitive function, and reduced inflammation.

Juniper

Juniper is a shrubby evergreen tree that grows in cooler climates worldwide. The bark is rough to the touch and contains high terpenes. These essential oils give juniper its characteristic flavor and scent. The tree is used for its wood, leaves, berries, and oil. Juniper products have many health benefits, including reducing inflammation, aiding digestion, and fighting anxiety and depression.

Kava Kava

Kava kava (Piper methysticum) is a shrub or small tree that grows up to 3 meters tall. Its branches are covered in sharp, pointed spines. The leaves are ovate-elliptical, 2 to 10 centimeters long and 1 to 5 millimeters wide, with deeply lobed margins. The white and bell-shaped flowers produce capsules that release the kava rootlets when opened. The rootlets grow into new plants.

There isn't one specific answer to this question as it depends on the person consuming it and their biology. Some people believe that kava interacts with the brain in a way that facilitates calmness and stress relief. Others say the herb has cognitive benefits, such as improving memory recall and concentration.

Some people even use it for its mood-boosting properties during anxiety or depression.

Kavalactones are compounds responsible for many of the purported benefits of kava kava consumption. The two most well-known substances are yangonin and kanavansine. For example, yangonin is thought to help lower blood pressure, while canavanine appears to have antidepressant effects. There's still much we don't know about the effects of kavalactones on the human body. Still, studies suggest they're likely safe — if taken in moderation.

Kola Nut

Kola nut is native to Africa and grows wild in central and eastern Africa. After being introduced to the Old World, kola nut **became popular in Arabia and Persia. Kola nuts were brought over to Europe by the Arab traders in the 7th century AD. Kola nuts are now grown in many parts of Africa. The best kola nuts are those from Nigeria, soaked in cold water for up to three weeks before being dried.**

Lady's Slipper

Lady's slipper (Cypripedium calceolus) is a plant native to North America and parts of Europe. It grows up to three feet tall with strap-like leaves and clusters of small, fragrant white flowers in late spring. The flower petals are extensions of the pistil, meaning they are non-functional and discarded when the flower blooms.

Lemon Balm

Lemon balm (Melissa officinalis) is a plant that has been used for centuries as a natural remedy for various ailments. It is native to North America and can be found in dry and wet habitats. Lemon balm is an erect, bushy shrub reaching up to 3 feet. The leaves are ovate-oblong, with serrated margins, and are covered in short, soft hairs.

Lemon Verbena

Lemon verbena is a member of the verbena family and is native to the eastern United States. Lemon Verbena is a hardy herb that can grow in various soils and climates. It has aromatic leaves and flowers that can be used in various food preparations, such as salads and soups. The leaves and flowers are also used to make tea, which can help improve circulation and relieve stress or anxiety.

Lemongrass

Native American herbs offer a wealth of benefits for the body and mind, making them an excellent addition to any health regimen. Lemongrass is one of the most popular native American herbs. Its many benefits include anti-inflammatory properties, improved mood and energy levels, and relief from headaches and congestion.

Licorice

Licorice (Glycyrrhiza glabra) is a flowering plant native to Eurasia and North Africa. The plant is noted for its sweet taste, from the glycyrrhizin compound in licorice root. Licorice has been used medicinally for centuries and has been shown to have a range of health benefits. These include reducing inflammation, improving blood sugar control, reducing high blood pressure, and supporting weight loss.

Lobelia

Lobelia is a succulent perennial herb with grass-like leaves and violet flowers. The species found in North America include L. cardinals, L. tenuifolia, and L. perennis, all of which have different benefits.

Lobelia has been used for centuries by American Indians as a medicinal herb. Studies have shown that it can treat colds, flu, bronchitis, asthma, and other respiratory problems. The plant is also believed to help improve moods and aid in relaxation. Some people also use it to reduce stress and anxiety.

Maca

Maca is a Peruvian root used for centuries as a source of energy and vitality. It is an adaptogen, meaning it helps the body resist stress. Maca also has antioxidant properties and can help improve fertility, libido, and male sexual function.

Maple

Maple is a hardy, deciduous tree that can grow up to 30 feet tall. The bark is scaly, and the leaves are ovate-oblong with serrated margins. The flowers are white and small, and the fruit is a small, round object that contains two seeds. The tree is native to North America but has been introduced to many other parts of the world.

Martin's Thistle

Martin's thistle (Cirsium arvense) is a member of the daisy family and native to central and eastern North America. The plant grows up to 3 feet tall, has purple flowers, and produces yellow seeds.

The main active ingredients in Martin's thistle are flavonoids, which are anti-inflammatory, antiviral, and antispasmodic. Additionally, the plant has been shown to help reduce cholesterol levels and protect the heart. In addition to its health benefits, Martin's thistle is also used for ornamental purposes.

Mayapple

Mayapple, also known as Indian hawthorn or mountain mayapple, is a shrubby herbaceous perennial plant in Berberidaceae. It is native to North America and can be found in many parts of the eastern and central United States and southern Canada. The plant grows to 1-3 m tall and has small, compound leaves that are elliptical or heart-shaped with serrated margins.

Milk Vetch

Milk vetch (Astragalus bisulfate) is a perennial herb that grows in North America's Great Plains and Rocky Mountains. Milk vetch has been used medicinally by Native Americans for centuries, and it is now being studied for its potential health benefits.

The root and leaves of milk vetch have been used to treat diarrhea, constipation, hay fever, bronchitis, and other respiratory problems. The roots also contain chemicals that help lower cholesterol levels and protect the heart. The stems and flowers of milk vetch are also used medicinally. The flowers are tea-like and sometimes used as a substitute for tea when traditional tea is unavailable or when people do not want to drink caffeinated beverages. The dried flowers can also be smoked as a form of recreational marijuana.

The bark of milk vetch has been used to treat pain, inflammation, fevers, headache, toothache, and other dental problems. The fruit of milk vetch is also eaten raw or cooked as a vegetable.

Milkweed

Milkweed is a plant that belongs to the daisy family. It grows in North America and Europe and is used as a natural remedy for various health problems. The plant contains a compound called milk, which has been found to have several health benefits. Some of these benefits are listed below.

Mint

Native American herbs are often used for medicinal purposes and have a long history of healing. Mint is one such herb, and its benefits are numerous.

Mint can help improve stomach function and relieve gas and bloating. It can also be used to treat colds, fevers, and headaches. In addition, mint is often used to boost the immune system.

Some other benefits of using mint include reducing inflammation, improving digestion, and promoting better circulation. While there are many different types of mint plants that will provide some of these benefits.

Mountain Hemlock

Mountain Hemlock (Conium maculatum) is a perennial herb that grows up to 2.5 meters tall. The plant has hairy stems and long, narrow leaves. The flowers are small and white, and the berries are purple or black. Mountain Hemlock has many benefits for Native Americans, including treating pain, improving blood circulation, reducing inflammation, and mitigating symptoms of fatigue and stress.

One of the most important uses for mountain hemlock is as a medicinal plant. The root can be used to treat pain relief and inflammation. At the same time, the leaves can improve blood circulation and treat symptoms of fatigue and stress. Additionally, mountain hemlock berries can be eaten as a food source or consumed as a medicine in tea form.

Mugwort

Mugwort (Artemisia vulgaris) is a wildflower that grows in temperate regions of the world. It is a member of the Artemisia genus. It is used as a herb to treat malaria, toothache, and other medical problems. Mugwort has also been traditionally used as a smoking herb for its euphoric properties.

Mullein

Mullein is a plant that grows in temperate climates around the world. The leaves and flowers of mullein are used to make a tea that is said to have many health benefits. Mullein can help improve circulation, relieve pain, and treat anxiety and depression. The tea can also help treat eczema, asthma, and other respiratory problems.

Nettle

Suppose you're considering natural remedies for your health concerns. In that case, it might be a good idea to look into herbs native to the United States. Some of the most popular American herbs include nettle, wild ginger, and dandelion.

Nettle is a plant that has been used as a medicinal herb for centuries. It is often used to treat joint pain, muscle aches and spasms, and other general symptoms. Additionally, nettle is known to help improve blood circulation and reduce inflammation.

Wild ginger is also a popular American herb. It is often used to treat pain relief, lower blood pressure, and improve digestion. Additionally, wild ginger can help boost the immune system and relieve symptoms of colds and flu.

Dandelion is another popular American herb. It is commonly used as a tea or tincture to treat kidney problems, respiratory problems, anxiety, and menstrual cramps. Additionally, dandelion can help reduce cholesterol levels and fight against cancerous cells.

Oak

Oak trees are tall and sturdy, with thick and rough bark. They are native to the Northern Hemisphere and can grow up to 160 feet tall. The leaves of an oak tree are broad and lobed, and they turn yellow-green in the fall. The acorns of an oak tree are a major food source for animals in the forests where they live and are also used for traditional medicines.

Olive Oil

Olive oil is a popular cooking oil found in many grocery stores. It is made from the fruit of the olive tree and has various health benefits.

Some benefits of consuming olive oil include: it's high in monounsaturated fats and antioxidants, which can help reduce the risk of heart disease, cancer, and other illnesses; it has anti-inflammatory properties; it provides satiety and reduces calories. Olive oil can also help decrease cholesterol levels, promote weight loss, improve cognitive function and memory recall, lower blood pressure, and relieve joint pain.

Oregano Grape

Oregano is a plant that grows in many parts of the world. It is a perennial herb that can be found growing in a variety of soils, including sandy soil. Oregano has been used for medicinal purposes for centuries and is now being studied for its health benefits. Some of the health benefits of oregano include reducing inflammation, fighting infection, and improving heart health.

Palo Santo

Many plants and herbs native to the United States have medicinal properties. Some of these plants are known as "palo santo" or "holy wood." Some of the most popular and well-known palo santo plants include sage, wormwood, rosemary, lavender, and thyme.

Some benefits of using palo santo for medicinal purposes include reducing inflammation, improving moods, boosting energy levels, treating anxiety and depression, and healing wounds. Many people also use palo santo to cleanse and purify their bodies.

Pasque flower

The Pasque flower (Aconitum napellus) is a plant that has a long history of use in traditional Chinese medicine and has been shown to have a wide range of health benefits. In particular, the pasque flower is thought to help ease anxiety, improving mood swings, and relieving stress. The pasque flower is believed to help improve circulation and reduce inflammation.

Passion Flower

Passionflower is a flowering plant that has been used medicinally for centuries. The plant has a long history of improving mood and promoting relaxation. Passionflower is also known to have health benefits, including reducing anxiety and depression, improving cognitive function, and increasing energy levels.

Partridgeberry

Partridgeberry is a small, dark purple-black fruit that grows on shrubs and trees in the eastern and central United States. The fruit is edible but not as well-known as other American native fruits, such as wild blueberries. The plant is used for its fruit, wood, and roots.

The benefit of partridgeberry is that it is a good source of vitamin C. It also contains antioxidants and other nutrients, like potassium and magnesium. These nutrients may help to protect cells from damage and may help to keep the body functioning properly.

Peppermint

Peppermint is a plant that originates from the Mediterranean region. It has been used medicinally for centuries and is now considered a safe and effective treatment for various ailments. The primary benefits of peppermint are that it is a natural anti-inflammatory, helps to improve mood swings, and can help to reduce anxiety levels.

Pine

Pine is a tall, slender tree found in the Northern Hemisphere. The needles are in bundles of two, and they are scale-like. The bark is rough to the touch and exudes a piney odor. The tree grows up to 20-30 m tall and has a diameter of 2-3 m. The needles are brown on the upper surface and white underneath. They have a distinctive fragrance that is often used in aromatherapy.

The tree is rich in sap which can be used for making syrup, turpentine, and wood tar. Wood is used to make bows, arrows, toys, furniture, and other items. Pine also provides shelter for deer, bears, squirrels, and porcupines.

Some of the benefits of using pine include reducing inflammation, treating arthritis and other joint pain, helping to improve respiratory health, boosting energy levels, aiding in weight loss efforts due to its high-calorie content, and improving skin health.

Plantain

Plantains are a type of plant that belongs to the banana family. They are native to tropical and subtropical regions and can be found in many different parts of the world. Plantains are frequently eaten as a vegetable, but they can also be used in savory dishes or as an accompaniment to other foods. Plantains are high in potassium, vitamin C, and dietary fiber. They are also a good source of magnesium, manganese, and vitamin B6.

Pleurisy Root

Pleurisy root is used to treat chest pain and other respiratory issues for centuries. It contains compounds that help relax the muscles in the chest, relieving symptoms such as coughing, shortness of breath, and rapid breathing. Additionally, pleurisy root is believed to help reduce inflammation of the lungs.

Poke

Poke is a traditional Native American dish made from fresh or frozen vegetables, meats, and occasionally fish. It can be served hot or cold and is often eaten as a side dish. Some of the most commonly used ingredients in poke include kale, Swiss chard, mustard greens, and collard greens; fruits such as mangoes, pineapple, lychee fruit, and grapefruit; and meats such as tuna steak, salmon fillet; chicken breast, and shrimp.

There are many benefits to incorporating some of the essential native American herbs and plants into your diet. These plants have been traditionally used for their medicinal properties. They have been found to support overall health and well-being. Some of the benefits of incorporating these plants into your diet include the following:

1) Supporting Healthy Digestion: Many of the indigenous plants used in poke are high in fiber which helps to promote healthy digestion. Fiber is important because it helps to keep your gastrointestinal system moving while helping to remove waste products from your body.

2) Promoting Heart Health: Several indigenous herbs and plants used in poke contain antioxidants that help to protect your heart against damage caused by free radicals. Free radicals are harmful molecules that can attack cell membranes and DNA, leading to diseases such as cancer. By including these plant-based antioxidants in your diet, you are providing important protection against heart disease.

Prickly Pear

A prickly pear is a shrub or small tree that can grow up to 10 feet tall. The fruit of the prickly pear is a round, spiny ball. The fruit is edible and can have many health benefits. Prickly pear fruit has high levels of vitamin C and B6 and magnesium and potassium. The fruit can also help improve digestion and reduce inflammation.

Prickly Pear Cactus

As the temperatures drop, many of us reach for warm drinks and comforting foods. One plant that is often overlooked but can be quite warming is the prickly pear cactus. These cacti are native to North America and have many benefits for humans and the environment.

Some of the benefits of using prickly pear cacti include:

1. The cactus can help add warmth to a room – especially during cold months when wood or other forms of heating may not be available.
2. The cactus has natural anti-inflammatory properties that can help ease pain and reduce inflammation in the body. This makes it a good choice for people with arthritis or joint pain.
3. The prickly pear cactus has antioxidants that help protect cells from damage, which may promote health and prevent diseases in the future.

Psyllium Seed Husk

Psyllium seed husks are a rich source of fiber and have numerous health benefits. They can help with weight loss, maintaining healthy blood sugar levels, managing heart disease risk factors, reducing inflammation, and aiding digestion. Psyllium husks are also commonly used as dietary supplements or to add bulk to foods.

Psyllium is a plant-based source of both soluble and insoluble fiber. Soluble fiber helps to reduce cholesterol levels and digestive problems. In contrast, insoluble fiber absorbs water and helps stabilize blood sugar levels by slowing the release of glucose into the bloodstream. In addition to these benefits, psyllium husks contain other minerals like magnesium, potassium, manganese, and copper, as well as antioxidants like lutein and zeaxanthin.

The most common use for psyllium husks is as a supplemental form of fiber. This is due to their high concentration of soluble fiber, which can help improve digestive function and reduce symptoms such as constipation or diarrhea. In addition, psyllium can help with weight loss since it increases satiety (the feeling of fullness after eating) and reduces caloric intake. Another benefit of using psyllium husks for supplemental fiber is that it can help reduce the risk of obesity and associated health problems such as heart disease or type 2 diabetes.

Purslane

Purslane is a plant commonly found in the wild and can be eaten as a vegetable. Researchers have studied the plant for years and have found many health benefits. Purslane has been shown to help improve blood pressure, cholesterol levels, and other heart conditions. It has also been shown to help prevent cancer and improve cognitive function.

Rabbit Tobacco

Some many native American herbs and plants have been used for centuries as remedies and sources of medicine. Some herbs, like rabbit tobacco, can provide physical and spiritual benefits to those who use them.

Rabbit tobacco is a plant that is indigenous to North America. It is a shrub or small tree that grows up to 6 feet tall. The leaves of the rabbit tobacco plant are triangular in shape and are covered in small, sharp needles.

The flowers of the rabbit tobacco plant are white and petal-less. They grow on short stalks near the base of the plant. The flowers contain an oil that is used to make smoking blends.

The root of the rabbit tobacco plant contains compounds that have medicinal properties. These compounds can help treat anxiety, depression, and chronic pain. In addition, the root of the rabbit tobacco plant can be used to treat asthma symptoms and varicose veins.

Some people believe that the herb rabbit tobacco has spiritual properties as well. It is said to help improve communication with spirit guides and other beings from other dimensions.

Ragleaf Bahia

Ragleaf Bahia is a West Indian herb that has long been used to treat various ailments. This herb has anti-inflammatory properties, which can help reduce swelling and inflammation. Additionally, ragleaf Bahia can help improve overall blood circulation. This herb is also thought to be beneficial for the respiratory system, as it can help decrease lung inflammation.

Red Clover

Red clover is a perennial plant that grows up to one meter tall. The leaves are alternately arranged and smooth to the touch. The flowers are small, white, and have five petals. They bloom from early spring to late summer and are pollinated by bees. Red clover is a good source of dietary fiber, protein, vitamins A, C, and E, potassium, magnesium, and iron.

Redroot

"Red Root" is a flowering plant native to North America. It is a part of the ginger family and has been used medicinally for centuries. The plant contains compounds that have anti-inflammatory properties that can help treat cramps and can improve heart health. Additionally, the plant can help lower blood pressure and improve circulation.

Rhodiola

Rhodiola Rosea is a perennial, aromatic plant that grows up to two meters tall. The root and stem are covered in small, white, daisy-like flowers. The leaves are large and curly, and the plant thrives in cold climates.

The root and stem contain rosavin, salidroside, and Scutellaria baicalensis extract (SBE), which have been shown to improve mood, cognitive function, energy levels, stress relief, and immune system health. These effects may be due to the plants' ability to improve central nervous system blood flow and oxygen delivery to the brain and other tissues.

Rhodiola can also help reduce anxiety and depression by improving communication between the brain's different parts. It has also been shown to improve memory function and vigilance.

Romero

Romero is a North American plant with a long history of use in traditional medicine. It is known for its healing properties, including helping to reduce inflammation and pain. Romero also has anti-inflammatory and antioxidant properties, making it a valuable remedy for various health concerns. Additionally, Romero helps to improve circulation and digestion.

Rooibos

Rooibos is a shrubby, perennial plant indigenous to South Africa. The leaves are arranged in whorls of three, and the red flowers are small and tube-shaped. Rooibos is used as a tea because of its high antioxidants, flavonoids, and caffeine levels. There are many reported health benefits to drinking rooibos tea, including reducing the risk of heart disease, dementia, Alzheimer's disease, stroke, cancerous tumors, and improved cognitive function.

Some other potential benefits of drinking rooibos include: aiding weight loss by stabilizing blood sugar levels, promoting better circulation, reducing inflammation; helping improve skin health; providing relief from anxiety and depression; improving sleep quality; and aiding in digestion.

Rose Hip

Rose hips are a key ingredient in many traditional Native American remedies. They have long been used as a food source. These sweet fruits contain vitamins A, C, and E, antioxidants, and minerals such as potassium, magnesium, zinc, and iron. Rose hips are also high in soluble fiber, which can help regulate blood sugar levels.

Some of the benefits of rose hip consumption include:

1. Rose hips are an excellent source of antioxidants that can help protect against cell damage and promote heart health.
2. Rose hips are also high in soluble fiber, which can help regulate blood sugar levels.
3. Rose hips provide Vitamin A, essential for healthy vision and immune system function.
4. Rose hips are a good source of magnesium which is important for maintaining nerve function and overall muscle health.

Sagebrush

Sagebrush (Artemisia tridentata) is a North American plant used for centuries as a remedy for various ailments. The plant contains several compounds that are believed to have health benefits, including reducing inflammation, promoting healing, and inhibiting the growth of cancer cells.

Saint John's Wort

Saint John's wort (Hypericum perforatum) is a perennial plant that grows up to one meter tall. It has purple flowers and red berries. Saint John's wort is a medicinal herb for treating various conditions, including depression, anxiety, and stress. Saint John's wort is also known to improve mood and relieve pain.

Saltbush

Saltbush is a succulent shrub that grows in dry, sandy soils. It is native to the Western United States and Eastern Canada. The plant has a long history of use by Native Americans for medicinal purposes. Saltbush can be used to treat a variety of health problems, including headaches, muscle pain, and arthritis. The plant also has anti-inflammatory properties.

Saltbush contains compounds that have antiviral and antiparasitic properties. The plant can also help to improve circulation and digestion. One of the benefits of using saltbush is that it is safe during pregnancy.

Sarsparilla

Sarsparilla (Smilax Officinalis) is a tall herbaceous perennial plant that grows to about 3 feet tall. The stem is woody at the base and covered with flat, smooth green leaves on the top and white below. Sarsparilla contains active ingredients such as flavonoids, tannins, saponins, and glycosides that provide medicinal benefits. The plant is used to relieve stomach cramps and gas, improve **digestion and stimulate appetite, as well as improve respiratory health.**

Savory

Savory is a flavor often associated with certain cuisines, such as Italian, French, and Mexican. In the United States, savory flavors are typically found in dishes like chicken cacciatore and beef stroganoff. Savory herbs and plants add complexity and depth of flavor to these dishes.

Saw Palmetto

Saw palmetto is a flowering shrub that is native to Florida and Georgia. The plant is well-known for its benefits in improving men's health, including reducing the risk of prostate cancer. Saw palmetto also has anti-inflammatory properties, which can help treat other conditions like arthritis. In addition to its medicinal properties, saw palmetto is also used as a natural dye and cosmetic ingredient.

The plant grows up to 3 feet tall and produces green or purple flowers. The fruit is an orange drupe that contains a kernel of crude oil that can be used for medicinal purposes. The bark and leaves of the saw palmetto are also used for cooking and cosmetics.

Senega Snakeroot

Senega Snakeroot is a plant used by Native Americans for centuries. The plant contains a compound called senega alkaloids, which are beneficial for health. Senega Snakeroot's benefits include improved immune system function, better blood circulation, and reductions in inflammation. In addition, Seneca snakeroot has anti-inflammatory properties and can help reduce pain from arthritis.

Senna Leaves

If you want to add some beneficial plant life to your garden but are unsure where to start, consider using Senna leaves. These leaves are high in antioxidants and have many health benefits. Here's a look at some of the benefits of using Senna leaves:

1. Help Reduce Inflammation: One of the primary benefits of using Senna leaves is that they help reduce inflammation. This is due to the presence of sennosides, which have anti-inflammatory properties.
2. Improve Digestion: Another benefit of using Senna leaves is that they improve digestion. This is because they contain tannins and other digestive aids.
3. Help Detoxify The Body: Finally, Senna leaves can also help detoxify the body by aiding in eliminating toxins and waste matter from the body.

Skunk Cabbage

Skunk cabbage (Symplocarpus foetidus) is a wild plant that grows in disturbed areas, such as abandoned fields and roadsides. It has extensive root systems that can spread extensively through the soil, so it's important to control its growth when using skunk cabbage in landscaping. The leaves and flowers are poisonous, but the root is not. The leaves are covered with a sticky secretion that contains toxins that cause constipation, diarrhea, and nausea when ingested. The flowers are also poisonous, but the stamen contains a sap that can be used in herbalism. Skunk cabbage is an excellent source of antioxidants and nutrients, including vitamin C, manganese, potassium, magnesium, and phosphorus.

Slippery Elm

Slippery elm (Ulmus rubra) is found throughout much of North America. It is often used as a natural remedy for arthritis, coughs, and respiratory problems. In addition to its medicinal properties, slippery elm is also known for its oil which has been used for centuries in traditional Native American remedies. The oil can be used topically or ingested and has been shown to have anti-inflammatory properties.

Smooth Upland Sumac

Smooth upland sumac (Rhus glabra) is a hardy shrub that grows up to 6 feet tall. The leaves are opposite, simple, and elliptical with a serrated margin. The flowers are small, white, and found in spikes at the ends of the branches. The fruit is a dry capsule that contains one to four black seeds. Smooth upland sumac is native to the Great Lakes region and can be found throughout most of Illinois.

The leaves have been used for medicinal purposes for centuries. Smooth upland sumac is known to be effective at treating skin conditions such as psoriasis, eczema, and dermatitis. The dried capsules can also be used as an insect repellent or tea to ease symptoms of arthritis or fever.

Stevia

One of the most popular plants in the world today is stevia. It is a perennial shrub or small tree with narrow leaves and sweet-tasting flowers. Stevia is native to tropical regions worldwide, but it was first discovered in South America. Today, stevia is grown commercially in several countries, including Taiwan, China, Paraguay, Brazil, and Uruguay.

Stevia has been used for centuries as a sweetener in Asia and South America. In recent years, it has also become more popular in North America. Stevia is 200 times sweeter than sugar and has no nutritional defects like other artificial sweeteners. Additionally, stevia contains zero calories, no gluten, and no sugar alcohol.

Some of the benefits of using stevia include:

It's calorie-free – so it can be used in place of sugar or other calorie-dense foods without worrying about weight gain or unhealthy calorie cravings;

It doesn't contribute to tooth decay – because it doesn't contain any sugar alcohols that can form plaque;

It's low glycemic index – meaning it won't raise blood sugar levels like regular sugar does, and

It's non-toxic – so it can be consumed by people of all ages without worry about side effects.

Stinging Nettle

Stinging nettle (Urtica dioica) is a common weed throughout North America. It has been used for centuries in traditional Medicine to treat various ailments, including pain, inflammation, and infection. Stinging nettle is also known for its stinging properties, which make it effective as a deterrent against predators and parasites.

Stinging nettle is an annual herb that grows up to 2 feet tall. The leaves are long and curved, with sharply pointy edges. The flowers are small and green, and the petals are smooth. The stinging hairs on the nettle plant are very sensitive to the touch, so be careful when handling it!

The root of the stinging nettle contains a compound called diosgenin, which is thought to be responsible for the plant's stinging abilities. Diosgenin can also be converted into an active drug called diosmin, which has anti-inflammatory properties.

Some benefits of using stinging nettle include:

1) It can help relieve pain and inflammation.

2) It can be a natural deterrent against predators and parasites.

3) It has anti-inflammatory properties that can help reduce symptoms associated with various diseases or injuries.

Stoneseed

Stoneseed is a perennial herbaceous plant in the daisy family Asteraceae. Native to North America, stoneseed grows in dry areas of the Great Plains and the Rocky Mountains. Stoneseed is a natural medicine traditionally used to treat asthma, bronchitis, heart disease, arthritis, varicose veins, and other conditions. The leaves and flowers are used in herbal remedies. Stoneseed can be purchased online or at health food stores.

Sumac

Sumac (Rhus typhina) is a shrubby tree or small bush found in North America and Eurasia. The fruit is a bright red drupe that can be used in drinks and sauces. The leaves are aromatic and have a pungent taste. Sumac is an astringent and has anti-inflammatory properties. It treats diarrhea, stomachaches, toothaches, colds, flu, and other infections. The bark is also used to treat skin conditions such as rashes, eczema, psoriasis, and boils. Sumac can also help relieve anxiety, depression, and headaches.

Sweetflag

Native American herbs and plants are valuable resources for health and well-being. Sweetflag (Asarum canadense), for example, is a popular herb used for medicinal purposes. The sweet flag has many benefits, including reducing inflammation, relieving pain, and fighting infections. Other native plants that have been used for medicinal purposes include elderberry (Sambucus canadensis), poke root (Phytolacca americana), and wild ginger (Asarum viride).

Suppose you want to improve your health by supplementing with natural herbs and plant extracts. In that case, some of the best options available are those found in Native American tradition. These plants offer potent remedies for common ailments and boast many other benefits, such as improved circulation, stronger immune systems, and deeper sleep. Here are five of the most essential Native American herbs and plants:

1) Sweetflag (Asarum canadense)

2) Poke Root (Phytolacca americana)

3) Elderberry (Sambucus canadensis)

4) Wild Ginger (Asarum viride)

5) Lavender (Lavandula angustifolia)

Sweetgrass

Sweetgrass is a grass found in many parts of the world, but it's especially prevalent on American Indian reservations. It is used for ceremonies and as a tea because of its sweet flavor and calming effects. There are many different types of sweetgrass, and some have more medicinal properties than others. Here are five of the most beneficial types:

Blue grama is a type of sweetgrass that is mostly used medicinally. It has anti-inflammatory properties and can help treat pain, indigestion, and anxiety.

Toothwort

Toothwort is a low-growing herb often found in moist areas throughout North America. The plant has leaves divided into lobes and a stem that can grow up to 2 feet tall. The flowers are small, white, and fragrant, and the seeds are small and black. The plant is an herbal remedy for various problems, including pain relief, fever reduction, and treating cold and flu symptoms. There are many different varieties of toothwort, each with specific benefits.

Toothwort is an effective treatment for pain relief. The plant contains chemicals called oligosaccharides that cause inflammation in the body. Oligosaccharides bind to receptors on nerve cells and block pain signals from reaching the brain. In addition to being an effective pain treatment, toothwort is believed to help reduce fever. The plant contains compounds that fight bacteria and reduce inflammation in the body.

Toothwort is also considered an antibacterial herb. One of the compounds in toothwort fights bacteria by disrupting their cell walls. This makes it difficult for bacteria to multiply and cause infection. Additionally, toothwort extract is effective in treating cold and flu symptoms. The antiviral properties of toothwort make it a useful treatment for these conditions.

Trumpet Honeysuckle

Trumpet honeysuckle (Lonicera sempervirens) is a hardy perennial vine that can grow up to 30 feet in length. The leaves are lance-shaped, and the flowers are trumpet-shaped, with white petals that alternate with dark sepals. Trumpet honeysuckle is native to North America and growing throughout most of the eastern United States, as well as in parts of Canada and Mexico. The plant is used medicinally by Native Americans, who use the juice from the flowers to treat colds, flu symptoms, indigestion, and other ailments. The flower's high levels of essential oil also make it an effective repellent against mosquitoes and other insects. Trumpet honeysuckle is a popular landscape plant due to its attractive flowers and vines.

Usnea

Usnea is a genus of lichen that can be found throughout the United States and Canada. Lichens are symbiotic organisms made up of an alga and a fungus, and Usnea is known for its antiviral properties. Lichens have been used by Native Americans for medicinal purposes for thousands of years, and they are still used today by many tribes.

There are over 100 species of Usnea, most of which have therapeutic benefits. Some examples of these benefits include antiviral, antibacterial, antifungal, anti-inflammatory, and antioxidant properties. Usnea can be taken as a supplement or used as a food additive.

Usnea has been shown to improve cognitive function and reduce human anxiety symptoms. It is also believed to protect the liver from damage caused by drugs and alcohol consumption.

Some common usnese supplements include usnese bark (Auricularia auricula-judge), usnese leaf (Lichenomphalia coronaria), usnese fruit (Lobaria muralis), and usnese sponges (Dictyocaulus filiformis).

Uva Ursi

Uva ursi is a plant that grows in the eastern and central United States. The plant is used as an herbal remedy to treat various medical conditions. Uva ursi contains compounds that have anti-inflammatory, anti-cancer, and antiseptic properties.

Venus's Slipper

In the United States, there are over 2,000 different species of plants that are considered essential to Native Americans. This is partly because of their historical and cultural connection to these plants. A few of these plants and herbs have been used for medicinal purposes for centuries, and many more have been used in ceremonies and rituals.

One such plant is Venus's slipper. This herb has several beneficial properties, including anti-inflammatory and antifungal agents. It can also help improve blood circulation and detoxify the body. In addition, Venus's slipper is an immune system booster and can help reduce anxiety and stress levels.

Water Birch

Water birch (Betula papyrifera) is a deciduous tree that can grow up to 30 feet tall. It has smooth, green leaves and small white flowers in late spring. The bark is rough and wrinkled, and the wood is light brown, hard, and strong. The water birch is native to eastern North America and can be found throughout much of Ontario and Quebec.

The water birch is valuable because it provides food, shelter, and materials for building products, medicines, tools, and other goods. Some of the benefits of water birch include:

-The water birch is a source of food. The nuts produced by the tree are high in protein and vitamin E. They are eaten fresh or roasted, or they can be used to make flour or oil.

-The water birch provides shelter for animals. Its smooth, green leaves provide shade from the sun during the day and keep the rain off crops at night. The tree also provides protection from wind and cold weather.

-The water birch is a source of materials for building products. Its hardwood can be used for furniture, tools, weapons, bridges, logging equipment, and other items.

-The water birch is a source of medicines. The bark contains tannins that have been used to treat various medical problems for centuries.

Watercress

Watercress, a curly dock or water spinach, is a leafy green plant native to North America. It can grow in wet streams, rivers, and lakes. Watercress leaves are high in vitamins A, C, and K, vitamin B6 and minerals such as potassium and magnesium.

Watercress leaves can be eaten fresh or dried in salads or as a garnish. It has anti-inflammatory properties and can help improve heart health. The herb also has cognitive benefits, promoting brain function and preventing Alzheimer's disease.

Western Hemlock

The western hemlock is a tall tree found in the mountainous regions of the Pacific Northwest. The bark is scaly and deeply furrowed, with large plates covering the trunk and branches. The leaves are ovate with pointed tips, and the flowers are white or light pink. The fruit is a cylindrical capsule containing one to four small seeds. There are many uses for western hemlock, both medicinally and spiritually.

The roots of western hemlock have been used to treat a variety of ailments for centuries, including fever, arthritis, and kidney problems. The bark can also be boiled to make a tea alleged to be anti-inflammatory and promote better breathing. Wood is also used to make furniture, tools, and other items.

Western hemlock has spiritual significance as well. Native Americans considered it a sacred plant because it was thought to contain powerful healing properties. They would use the sap from the branches to seal wounds or apply it to burns as an ointment. Today, some people use western hemlock juice or tincture as a natural remedy for anxiety, depression, ADD/ADHD, seizures, fatigue, sinus problems, and other health issues.

Western Skunk Cabbage

Some of the most commonly used herbs and plants in Native American Medicine are western skunk cabbage, wild ginger, dandelion, garlic, and yarrow. Western skunk cabbage (Symplocarpus foetidus) is a member of the Brassica family and is native to North America. The herb has been used for centuries to treat various issues, including heart problems, respiratory problems, arthritis pain, gastrointestinal issues, mental health conditions, and skin issues.

The benefits of western skunk cabbage include:

-The plant is anti-inflammatory and helps reduce swelling and pain from arthritis

-It can help improve breathing by increasing airflow and decreasing inflammation

-It can help improve digestion by reducing inflammation in the gut and promoting better absorption of nutrients

-It can help improve mental health by reducing anxiety and depression symptoms

Western Stoneseed

Western stoneseed (Astragalus membranaceus) is a perennial herb growing up to 1.5 meters tall with white, pink, or yellow flowers. The root is a medicinal plant, and the leaves are an important part of the Native American diet. Flowers have been found to contain high levels of minerals such as potassium, magnesium, calcium, iron, and zinc. Some studies have also shown that flowers can help improve blood circulation and reduce inflammation. The leaves can be eaten fresh or dried and are often used in soups or stews.

White Pine

Overview and benefits of some essential native American herbs and plants

Native Americans have long used herbs for medicinal purposes, and their knowledge of herbal Medicine is still being studied. Some of these plants are now considered essential to the health of people and wildlife. Here are a few of the most important herbs and plants that Native Americans use:

White pine (Pinus strobus)

This tree is known for its anti-inflammatory properties, which make it a good choice for treating arthritis. It's also been used to treat respiratory problems, anxiety, depression, and nausea.

Birch (Betula papyrifera)

Native Americans used birch bark to make birch beer and wine. The tree is also high in beta-carotene, which helps prevent eye disease and skin cancer.

The leaves and bark can also be used as a natural treatment for irritated eyes, sinusitis, toothache, acne, eczema, psoriasis, burns, skin infections including mono and pneumonia, and more.

White Sage

White sage, Salvia apiana, is one of the most common and widely used herbs in Native American Medicine. The leaves and branches treat various conditions, including headaches, anxiety, menstrual cramps, toothaches, and colds. The plant is also known for its anti-inflammatory properties. It has been used to treat arthritis and other joint pain.

Wild Buckwheat

Wild buckwheat is a common wildflower that can be found throughout North America. This flower is native to Eurasia and is thought to have been domesticated by the ancient Greeks. Wild buckwheat contains high levels of protein, fiber, and antioxidants. The flowers are edible and can be used in salads or as a standalone grain.

Wild Ginger

Wild ginger (Zingiber officinale) is a plant that grows in the United States, Canada, and parts of Europe. The root and stem of wild ginger are used to make Medicine.

The benefits of using wild ginger include reducing inflammation, treating pain, and improving circulation. Some people also use it to improve cognitive performance and lower blood pressure.

Wild ginger can be purchased online or at health food stores. It should be stored in a cool, dark place.

Wild Ham

Wild ham, also known as berry-of-the-wool, is one of the most common American herbs and plants. This plant often grows in disturbed areas such as fields and along roadsides. The fruit of the wild ham plant is an edible purple berry, although some people find it to be sour.

The various parts of the wild ham plant have many beneficial properties. The roots are used to make Medicine, while the leaves and young shoots are used as an additive in food or drinks. The bark has also been used to treat various ailments, such as skin conditions and infections. In addition to these benefits, the fruit can be eaten raw or cooked, providing nutrients such as vitamins A and C.

Wild Lettuce

Wild lettuce, or lamb quarters, is an annual plant that grows in many different parts of the United States. It has a long history of use as a medicinal herb, and it is currently being studied for its potential health benefits.

Wild lettuce is a member of the Asteraceae family, which contains dozens of plants with medicinal properties. The leaves and flowers of wild lettuce can be used to make tea, tincture, or extract. The leaves also make a salad dressing called "wild balsamic vinaigrette."

Some of the benefits of consuming wild lettuce include: reducing inflammation, boosting the immune system, regulating blood sugar levels, fighting cancer cells, and helping to reverse age-related declines in cognitive function.

Willow

The willow tree is a common sight in many parts of North America, from the high elevations of the Rocky Mountains to humid rainforests. The wood from the willow tree is used for various purposes, including building materials and furniture.

There are many benefits to using willow products in your life. Willow bark is an effective natural treatment for fever, inflammation, and other medical conditions. The leaves and branches of the willow tree can be used as a source of food, Medicine, and shelter.

The willow tree grows quickly and is versatile enough to be used in various settings. It can be planted near homes or businesses to provide shade and reduce air conditioning costs or used in parks and nature preserves as a source of wildlife habitat.

Witch Hazel

Witch hazel (Hamamelis virginiana) is a shrub or small tree that can grow up to 8-12 feet tall. It has sparsely hairy leaves on the upper surface and scale-like underneath. The flowers are white, and the fruit is a brown pod. Witch hazel is used for treating skin problems, including dryness, inflammation, itchiness, and sunburn.

Some other benefits of witch hazel include anti-inflammatory, antiviral, antimicrobial, and detoxifier. It can also help improve circulation and reduce swelling. Additionally, it has been used to treat pain relief, reducing stress levels and tension headaches.

Wormwood

Wormwood (Artemisia absinthium), also known as mugwort, is a plant that grows wild in many parts of the world. Indigenous peoples in North America and Europe have used wormwood for medicinal purposes for centuries. Wormwood has been used to treat colds, flu, tuberculosis, and other respiratory infections. It can also be used to reduce inflammation and help relieve pain.

Wormwood is often considered a potent herbal remedy. However, like all herbs, they should be used with caution and only under the guidance of a healthcare professional. Some potential side effects of taking wormwood include dizziness, drowsiness, and confusion. If pregnant or breastfeeding, speak with your doctor before using wormwood supplements.

Yan Cao

Yan Cao, known by the scientific name Cynanchum wilfordii, is a North American plant. It is a member of the mint family and grows in moist areas near streams and rivers. The leaves and flowers are used medicinally and are also reported to be edible.

Yarrow

Yarrow (Achillea millefolium) is a common herbaceous flowering plant found in temperate areas of the world. The leaves are opposite, ovate to lance-shaped, and serrated on the margins. The flowers are small, blue or purple, with 5 petals. Yarrow is an important medicinal plant and has been used for centuries to treat a variety of health conditions.

The leaves and flowers of yarrow can be used to make teas and tinctures. The leaves can be dried and subsequently brewed as tea or added to herbal remedies as a flavoring agent. The flowers can also be made into capsules or infused oil for topical use. The root of the yarrow plant can be used in various ways, including as a tonic, bitter extract, emetic, and diuretic.

Yellow Dock

The yellow dock (Veronica Anagallis) is a flowering plant native to the eastern United States. The roots of the yellow dock can be used to make a tea that is said to have medicinal benefits. Some benefits of yellow dock include reducing inflammation, improving digestion, and treating various diseases and conditions.

Yellow Gentian

Many beneficial plants native to North America can be used for medicinal purposes. One of these herbs is the yellow gentian (Gentiana lutea), which has been used medicinally by Native Americans for centuries.

The yellow gentian is a perennial plant that grows up to 2 feet tall. The leaves are alternate, 1 to 3 inches long, with serrated edges. The flowers are bell-shaped with bright yellow petals and reddish-brown spots on the inside of the petals.

The root system of the yellow gentian is a diuretic and antioxidant, providing benefits for kidney health and overall strength. The herb has also been used to treat fever, gastrointestinal problems, anxiety, arthritis, and other conditions.

Yerba Mate

Yerba Mate is a traditional tea made from the leaves of the yerba mate plant. Yerba mate is popular in South America and is considered a social beverage. It has many beneficial properties, including caffeine and antioxidant activity.

Many herbalists believe that yerba mate can improve cognitive function and circulation. Additionally, yerba mate Contains polyphenols and catechins, which have anti-inflammatory properties. These compounds help reduce stress levels and support a healthy mind and body. Some studies also show that yerba mate can reduce anxiety and depression symptoms.

Yerba Sant

Yerba Sant is a popular and healthy tea made from the leaves and flowers of several different plants, including sage, yarrow, mint, peppermint, and calendula.

Some common benefits of drinking yerba sant tea include improved circulation, better mental clarity and focus, reduced stress levels, improved digestion, and more. Some people also use it as a natural remedy for anxiety and depression.

Some of the specific plants that are used to make yerba sant include sagebrush (Artemisia tridentata), goldenseal (Hydrastis Canadensis), lambsquarters (Chenopodium album), mullein (Verbascum thapsus), peppermint (Mentha piperita) and calendula (Calendula officinalis).

Yucca

Many plants have been used by native Americans for medicinal purposes. Yucca is one such plant. Yucca has a long history of use as a medicinal herb by many different cultures. Yucca contains compounds that have many health benefits, including reducing inflammation and pain, improving nerve function, and treating respiratory issues.

Yucca has been used to treat various conditions, including respiratory issues, inflammation, and pain. It is effective in reducing both chronic and acute inflammation. Studies were done on animals it was found to be effective in reducing pain caused by various injuries and diseases. Additionally, it was found to help improve nerve function and function overall.

Yucca can also be used in natural remedies for respiratory issues such as asthma. Studies done on asthma animals showed it was effective in reducing symptoms and improving lung function. Additionally, it helps reduce congestion and improve breathing overall.

Zizzi Aurea

There are many benefits to incorporating native American herbs and plants into your health and wellness routine. Some of the most notable include:

1. Native Americans have used these plants for centuries to improve their health and well-being.

2. They have a wide range of properties that can help support overall well-being, including anti-inflammatory, antiseptic, detoxifying, and analgesic effects.

3. These plants also support the immune system since they contain natural antibiotics and antioxidants.

4. Some plants can also improve mood and cognitive function thanks to their naturally occurring compounds, such as flavonoids and terpenes.

Book 5:
Native American Essential Oils Vol 1

Chapter 1: An Overview Of Essential Oils

Essential oils are all the rage these days, and for a good reason. These tiny ingredients offer a wealth of benefits for both the body and mind, making them a popular choice for personal care products and herbal remedies. But just what are essential oils, and what do they do? This section will provide an overview of essential oils and their many benefits. We will also provide tips on how to use them safely and effectively. So, whether you're looking to improve your health or find new ways to relax, read on for all the details you need about essential oils!

What Are Essential Oils?

Essential oils are a type of plant-derived oil. They are extracted from aromatic plants by steam distillation. The most common plants used to extract essential oils are lavender, chamomile, thyme, and lemon balm.

There are over 100 different essential oils that have been documented and used in perfumes, soaps, lotions, supplements, food flavorings, and more. Some well-known essential oils include lavender oil, peppermint oil, tea tree oil, and ginger oil.

What Are The Benefits Of Essential Oils?

There are many benefits to using essential oils, both internally and externally. Some of the benefits include:

- Essential oils can be helpful for headaches and migraines.
- They can be helpful for respiratory problems, including asthma and bronchitis.
- They are also beneficial for skin conditions such as eczema and psoriasis.
- They can help to improve moods and feelings of well-being.
- They can help relieve stress and anxiety.

Things To Keep In Mind Before Using Essential Oil

If you're looking to add some essential oils to your aromatherapy arsenal, there are a few things to keep in mind. First, make sure you buy quality oils—you don't want any diluted or chemicals added. Second, be careful when using them; essential oils can be extremely potent and should be used in moderation. Finally, always test out a new oil on a small area before using it on larger areas.

How Do You Choose The Right Essential Oil For You?

When choosing essential oils, choosing the right oil for your needs is important. There are many different types of essential oils, and each works best in specific situations.

To find the right oil for you, start by reading what the oil is used for. Essential oils are often used as supplements or remedies, so it is important to understand their uses before purchasing them. Additionally, research the properties of each oil before making a purchase.

Some essential oils can be harmful if ingested or in contact with the skin. Always be sure to follow the safety guidelines for each type of oil when using it.

It is also important to consider your climate when selecting an essential oil. Some oils work better in warmer climates, while others work better in cooler climates. Check the weather forecast before purchasing any essential oils to ensure they will work in your particular environment.

What Are Some Dangers Of Using Essential Oils Incorrectly?

There are many dangers of using essential oils incorrectly. Some common problems include toxic exposure, skin irritation and inflammation, and hormone disruption. Toxic exposure can happen when essential oils are mixed with other chemicals or applied directly to the skin. Skin irritation and inflammation can be caused by too much oil or by using oils that are not safe for topical use. Hormone disruption can occur if essential oils are taken in high doses or applied to areas with a lot of hair growth.

Essential Oils And Native American People

Essential oils are extracted from plants and have been used by people for centuries. The plants from which essential oils are extracted can be found worldwide. One of the most popular places to find essential oils is in Native American cultures.

Native Americans have used essential oils for various purposes for thousands of years. Some uses include treating infections, preventing disease, boosting moods, and helping with relaxation. Many of these uses are still being studied today and much more likely remain unknown.

Several different essential oil blends can be used for various purposes. It is important to consult with a professional before using any essential oil to ensure that it is safe and effective for your specific needs.

Chapter 2: The Benefits Of Using Oils

Helps Relieve Headaches

Essential oils are natural remedies used for centuries to help relieve headaches. The most common essential oils used to treat headaches include lavender, peppermint, and lemon.

When applied topically to the scalp, lavender oil is excellent for treating headaches because it is a relaxant. Peppermint oil also has analgesic properties, which can help reduce pain and inflammation. Lemon oil is also effective in relieving headaches because it has anti-inflammatory properties.

Helps Reduce Nausea

When it comes to helping reduce nausea, the key is to find oils that work best for you. Lavender, ginger, and peppermint are some of the most common essential oils used to help with nausea.

Each oil has its own specific benefits when it comes to reducing nausea. Lavender oil is known to be soothing and effective at decreasing anxiety and stress levels. Ginger oil can help improve digestive function and fight nausea by stimulating the appetite. Peppermint oil is also helpful in fighting nausea because it helps to stimulate the central nervous system.

Finding an oil that works best for you is key to reducing nausea. However, using a variety of oils together can also increase their overall effectiveness.

Helps Reduce Inflammation

There are many benefits to using essential oils, including reducing inflammation.

One study found that the use of lavender oil may help reduce inflammation in the eyes. This is likely due to the anti-inflammatory properties of the oil.

Other essential oils that help reduce inflammation include ginger, tea tree, and thyme. These oils have antibacterial and antifungal properties, which may help reduce the growth of bacteria and fungi that can cause inflammation.

Helps Improve Your Sleep

Essential oils can help improve your sleep. Here are some of the wide benefits:

1. Essential oils can help you relax and fall asleep faster. Some essential oils, like lavender, can help reduce anxiety and stress levels, making them ideal for people who struggle to get a good night's sleep. Others, like peppermint, promote relaxation and help you sleep quickly.

2. Essential oils can also improve your mood and energy level during the day. Some essential oils, such as lavender and lemon balm, effectively reduce stress levels and promote a more positive outlook on life. Combined with other natural remedies like exercise, these essential oils may help you maintain better mental health throughout the day.
3. Essential oils can also improve your sleeping habits in the long run. By gradually introducing essential oils into your nightly routine, you may find that they promote better sleep hygiene, which could lead to longer bouts of restful slumber.

Reduces Anxiety and Pain

One of the most common uses for essential oils is as an aromatherapy remedy for reducing anxiety and pain. In studies examining the use of essential oils for anxiety relief, it has been found that certain essential oils (such as lavender) can help reduce symptoms such as nervousness, stress, racing heart rates, and sleeplessness. Additionally, some essential oils (like tea tree) are known to be effective at helping to fight infection and relieve pain.

Helps Reduce Migraine

According to the Cleveland Clinic, headaches are one of the most frequent pain-related health concerns, impacting up to 75% of individuals globally. According to Johns Hopkins Medicine, migraine, a more severe kind of headache, affects about 12% of individuals in the United States. As the Cleveland Clinic points out, headaches are a major cause of absenteeism from work and school. They can contribute to feelings of anxiety and sadness.

Some people seek relief from essential oils such as peppermint, and there is some very limited study on its value for headaches. According to one review, applying peppermint oil superficially to the head and temples can help relieve headaches. This could be because of menthol, the main active element in peppermint. According to an uncontrolled investigation of 25 individuals that investigated migraine pain severity after applying a 6 percent menthol gel to the pain site, menthol offers a cooling sensation that is hypothesized to have an analgesic (pain alleviating) effect. Those that used the gel for migraines observed significant reductions in headache intensity two hours after application.

Helps Balance Out Hormones

Hormone essential oils can help balance your estrogen, progesterone, cortisol, thyroid, and testosterone levels.

Some oils, such as clary sage, geranium, and thyme, assist regulate estrogen and progesterone levels, aiding with diseases such as infertility, PCOS, PMS, and menopause symptoms.

According to a 2017 study published in Neuroendocrinology Letters, geranium and rose can impact the salivary levels of estrogen in women. This may benefit people experiencing menopausal symptoms caused by decreased estrogen secretion.

Certain oils have been shown to lower cortisol levels, which can help improve your mood, minimize depression symptoms, and enhance testosterone levels, improving a man's libido.

Boosts Skin Condition

Using essential oils on your skin and in hair and beauty products is a natural and effective approach to maintaining your personal care routines without using products containing chemicals and hydrogenated oils. Essential oils can help to soothe irritated skin, minimize aging signs, alleviate acne, protect your skin from sun damage, and thicken your hair.

Research published in Evidence-Based Complementary and Alternative Medicine states that "at least 90 essential oils are suggested for dermatological usage, with at least 1,500 combinations." The capacity of these oils to fight microorganisms that cause dermatological diseases gives them their skin advantages.

Oils can also help with inflammatory skin problems such as dermatitis, eczema, and lupus, improve the overall appearance of your skin, and aid in wound healing.

There have also been numerous studies that show essential oils to be beneficial for hair development. A 2015 study looked at the effects of rosemary oil on patients with androgenetic alopecia, or male or female pattern baldness.

Patients were randomly given either rosemary oil or minoxidil (a drug routinely used to treat hair loss) for a six-month treatment period. At the six-month mark, researchers discovered that both groups had a considerable rise in hair count. They also found that the minoxidil group experienced higher scalp itchiness.

Lowers Body Toxicity

By stimulating the detoxification of your house and body, essential oils can help minimize toxins. We all inhale and swallow various chemicals and environmental contaminants, which can harm our hearts, brains, and overall health.

Some oils act as mild diuretics, enhancing urine output and detoxifying. According to research, some oils improve digestion and detoxify toxins that accumulate within the body.

Detoxifying oils can help flush out these pollutants while also cleaning the air in your house. In fact, unlike most chemical-laden house cleaning products, essential oils may organically clean your home by removing hazardous bacteria and contaminants.

Grapefruit, orange, lemon, lemongrass, eucalyptus, and cinnamon are essential oils for lowering toxins in your home or workplace.

Chapter 3: How To Use Essential Oils

What Is Aromatherapy?

Aromatherapy uses essential oils to improve mood, relaxation, and well-being. Essential oils are natural extracts that come from plants. They have been used for centuries to treat a variety of ailments. There are many different types of essential oils, each with unique benefits.

Some of the most common essential oils used in aromatherapy include lavender, chamomile, peppermint, frankincense, and myrrh. These oils can be inhaled or applied topically to the skin. When used topically, essential oils can be mixed with a carrier oil (such as jojoba oil) to form a cream or lotion.

Aromatherapy has been shown to have various benefits for people of all ages. It can help relieve anxiety and depression, reduce stress levels, improve sleep quality, and more.

When using essential oils in aromatherapy, it is important to know your body chemistry and health conditions. Some people are sensitive to certain chemicals found in essential oils, so it is important to consult with a healthcare professional before using them therapeutically.

Through Steam Inhalation

Steam inhalation is a great way to use essential oils. You can diffuse or inhale the oils directly from a steam inhaler. Diffusing the oils helps to spread them around the room while inhaling them directly allows you to get more of the scent in your nose.

Using An Essential Oil Diffuser

Suppose you're looking for an easy and convenient way to add essential oils to your everyday routine. In that case, a diffuser is a perfect option. Diffusers work by dispersing the oil into the air, which makes it easy to inhale and use.

To get started, figure out what type of diffuser you want. There are ultrasonic diffusers, which use high-frequency sound waves to break up the oil molecules and disperse them into the air. This diffuser is best for those who want a light misting of the essential oil rather than full-on diffusion; it also has a shorter operating time than other diffusers.

Consider an electronic diffuser if you're looking for something with more power. These devices use electrical currents to heat the oil, breaking down its molecular structure and dispersing it into the air. They tend to be more powerful than ultrasonic or heat-based diffusers and have longer operating times.

Once you've determined what type of diffuser you need, gather your supplies: distilled water, essential oils (either bought pre-mixed or diluted yourself), and your diffuser. Add 2 teaspoons of distilled water per cup of essential oil(or desired dosage), mix well, and pour into your diffuser. Turn on your machine and wait for it to warm before adding your oils.

There are many different ways to use essential oils in our daily lives, so experiment until you find some techniques that work best for you. Adding a diffuser to your routine can make using essential oils more convenient and enjoyable.

Using Essential Oils In Bath

If you're looking to add a little more zing to your bath time routine, essential oils may just be what you need. Many of these oils are known for their therapeutic properties and can help relax the mind and body.

Here are four ways to use essential oils in your bath:

1. Add a drop or two of oil to the soap for an added relaxation layer. Lavender is a great choice for this because it has been shown to promote a sense of calmness and peace.

2. Add oil to the water before bathing for added invigorating properties. Tea tree oil is a popular pick because it is thought to be antibacterial and antiseptic, helping keep your skin healthy while you soak.

3. Add a few drops of oil directly to the hot bathtub for a soothing effect. Chamomile, lavender, and ginger are all good choices here because they improve sleep quality and relieve stress, headaches, and pain.

4. Use essential oils as aromatherapy in your bedroom at night before bedtime for enhanced relaxation and improved sleep quality. A few drops of lavender, chamomile, or rosemary work wonders here!

Using Topically

Because essential oils are fat soluble, they are quickly absorbed by the skin. A popular technique to use essential oils is to apply them to your skin for absorption - but never directly on the skin. It is always combined and diluted with a carrier oil like sweet almond oil or apricot kernel oil.

If skin sensitivity is an issue, ALWAYS dilute your essential oil with a common neutral carrier oil (also known as base oil) before application. Carrier oils are primarily cold-pressed oils that do not evaporate like essential oils. Still, they can go rancid in ways that essential oils do not. To avoid allergic responses, your carrier oil selection will be influenced by your preferences for scent, texture, and sensitivities. Popular carrier oils include coconut oil, sweet almond oil, jojoba oil, avocado oil, sunflower oil, and grape seed oil.

Essential oils are commonly applied to the skin on the wrists, temples, feet, and ears.

Inhaling The Fragrance

You can cautiously inhale your essential oils. Open the bottle of essential oils, place a few drops against your nose or on a tissue, and take a deep breath to inhale and enjoy. When using a new essential oil for the first time, use only one drop to ensure no reaction or sensitivity to the oil.

As you inhale, try to maintain your breath calm. Check to see if it gets trapped in the body or flows in and out easily. A deep breath is not the same as a sniff. Slow, deep breaths will signal to your head that your body needs to relax, and your entire body will follow. Your body and mind are not different entities, and often deceiving the body into relaxing first will put the mind in a position to rest.

You are aware that breathing is essential to your survival. Deep breathing can benefit one's health and well-being when it is simple, natural, and required. When you are feeling anxious, it is one of the simplest and most efficient techniques to calm down and regain your composure. The secret is deep belly breathing. And when combined with aromatherapy via essential oils, such breathing will assist in balancing our nervous system and reduce the amount of stress in our lives.

Chapter 4: How To Store Essential Oils

When stocking up on essential oils, it's important to store them correctly. Not only will improperly stored oils give you unpleasant smells, but they can also be dangerous. This section will outline the best ways to store essential oils and help you avoid common mistakes. From properly storing oils in a cool, dark place to keeping them away from heat and light, this section has everything you need to keep your essential oils safe and effective.

What Causes Essential Oils To Breakdown?

Essential oils are made up of various plant-based molecules and can be susceptible to breaking down over time. Climate control, light exposure, air pollution, and other environmental factors can all contribute to the gradual breakdown of essential oils.

Some common causes of essential oil breakdown include:

- Exposure to air conditioning or heating systems: Air conditioning and heating systems often cause the temperature and humidity in a room to fluctuate, which can damage essential oils. Over time, this can lead to the oils breaking down into smaller molecules more easily absorbed by the air.

- Heat exposure: Sunlight and heat also play a role in the deterioration of essential oils. When heated above 150 degrees Fahrenheit, certain chemical compounds within the oil will start to break down. This can accelerate the process of oxidation, which is how essential oils lose their therapeutic properties.

- UV radiation: Ultraviolet (UV) radiation is known for its ability to damage skin cells and tissues. This type of radiation also damages essential oil molecules, which can lead to their degradation over time.

Things To Keep In Mind While Storing

Always Make Sure To Keep Them Away From Light And Heat

When storing essential oils, always make sure to keep them away from light and heat. Exposure to either can damage the oil's delicate properties. If you are traveling with your essential oils, pack them in a cool and dark place.

Using Wooden Storage Boxes

Storage boxes made of wooden materials are perfect for storing essential oils because they are natural and do not emit harmful chemicals. Wooden storage boxes can store different essential oils, such as lavender oil, peppermint oil, and eucalyptus oil.

Always follow the manufacturer's instructions when storing essential oils in wooden boxes. Some essential oils, such as lavender, can be stored at a low temperature. In contrast, others, like peppermint, can be stored at a higher temperature. You should also remember that some essential oils, such as lavender, may release a scent when stored in a wooden box.

Using Fabric Storage Boxes

When storing essential oils, you may consider fabric boxes appropriate for the type of oil. A box made of thin cardboard will be sufficient if the oil is a light oil, such as rose or lavender. A stronger box made of wood or metal is needed for heavier oils, such as peppermint or ginger.

When selecting a fabric storage box, it is important to consider the size and shape of the oil. Some oils may fit into a small container, while others require a larger container. It is also important to decide on the level of protection the oil will need. A box with a tight-fitting lid will provide more protection than one with a loosely fitting lid.

Storing In Your Kitchen Cabinets

The kitchen is one of the most important rooms in your home and one of the most overlooked. Not only does a cluttered kitchen make cooking difficult, but it can also lead to a messier home overall. That's why it's important to take the time to properly store your essential oils, so they're easy to find and use when you need them.

When storing essential oil bottles, always keep them upright, so the oil doesn't spill out. Also, label each bottle with its corresponding scent(s). You can do this by writing the scent name on a piece of paper and tucking it inside the bottle or using a small sticker that you can place on top.

When it comes to storage containers, choose airtight and glass-lined ones, so the oils don't discolor or become rancid. It's also important to store your oils in a cool, dark place where they won't be exposed to sunlight or heat. If you have questions about properly storing essential oils, ask your Essential Oil Guide!

Storing In Airtight Bottles

Essential oils should be stored in a cool, dark, and airtight location to retain their potency. Areas not ideal for storage include direct sunlight, extreme temperatures, and high humidity.

It is important to keep the bottles tightly sealed when storing essential oils to avoid leakage and contamination. Some people prefer to store their essential oils in glass bottles. In contrast, others opt for plastic containers because they are more airtight. It is also helpful to rotate your stock periodically so that you're not using old or contaminated oil.

Storing In Refrigerators

When storing essential oils in a refrigerator, ensure the bottles are tightly closed and placed on a level surface.

Do not store oils in the freezer. They will become clumpy and will not last as long. If you're traveling with your essential oil stash, pack them in a cool, airtight container.

Storing In a Cool And Dark Place

Essential oils should always be stored in a cool, dark place to maintain potency. This means the bottle should be stored in the refrigerator if you use it within 2 weeks and in a cool, dark cabinet if it is longer than two weeks. If not using the oil immediately, store it in a small glass container with a lid that can be tightly closed. Pour a little oil into your hand and smell it; if it doesn't have an odor, put it back into the bottle. Make sure to label your bottles with the oil's name and the date they were filled.

Check The Expiration Date Before Buying

When storing your essential oils, the expiration date must be kept in mind. Essential oils are susceptible to oxidation and deterioration if kept beyond their recommended expiration dates. Oils that have been stored properly will generally have a longer shelf life than oils that have not been stored properly.

Some tips for proper oil storage include keeping oils in the dark glass or stainless-steel containers and store away from heat, light, and moisture. It is also important to check the expiration date before purchasing oil to know how long it will last.

Book 6:
Native American Essential Oils Vol 2

Chapter 1: List Of All Crucial Essential Oils

There are many benefits to using essential oils in the home and for our health. One of the most popular essential oils is lavender. In this section, we will explore the uses of lavender oil and some of its key benefits. From calming anxiety to promoting relaxation, this essential oil has many benefits that can be enjoyed internally and externally. We will also explore common ways to use lavender oil, from topical applications to diffusers. So if you're looking for an essential oil that can offer various benefits, look no further than lavender!

Cedarwood Oil

Cedarwood oil has a sweet, woodsy, and spicy scent. It has been used for centuries as a natural remedy for various ailments, including cedarwood oil for acne. Cedarwood oil is also reputed to help balance emotions and promote relaxation.

Lavender Oil

Lavender oil is a popular essential oil used in aromatherapy and for its relaxing effects. It is derived from the flowers of the lavender plant and has a sweet, herbal scent. Lavender oil can be used to treat a variety of conditions, including anxiety, stress, depression, and insomnia.

Sweet Grass Oil

Sweetgrass oil is an essential oil derived from the flowering tips of various types of grass. It has a warm, grounding scent that promotes relaxation and stress relief. Sweetgrass oil is also used to treat anxiety, depression, and other mental health issues.

Sage Oil

Native American sage oil is a potent essential oil used for centuries to promote health and well-being. This oil is derived from the sage plant's leaves, stems, and flowers. It is often used as a natural remedy for various conditions, including anxiety, depression, chronic pain, and respiratory issues.

Sage oil also effectively treats skin problems such as blemishes and eczema. Some people also use it to treat other conditions, such as headaches, asthma, and menstrual cramps.

Peppermint Oil

Peppermint oil is a common essential oil that has been used for centuries by indigenous people all over the world. It is abundant in menthol and has a cooling effect on the body. Peppermint oil can be used to relieve anxiety, headaches, and nausea. It can also be used as an additive to massage oil or mouthwash.

Eucalyptus Oil

Eucalyptus oil (also called blue gum oil) is a natural, essential oil obtained from the leaves and branches of the eucalyptus tree. The oil treats various infections and respiratory problems, including colds, bronchitis, and asthma. It can also be used to soothe skin irritation and inflammation.

Rosemary Oil

Rosemary oil is a popular essential oil used for centuries by Native Americans. Rosemary is a rich source of antioxidants, including beta-carotene, lutein, and zeaxanthin. It is also effective in treating respiratory problems and inflammation.

Cypress

Cypress essential oil can strengthen gums, prevent infections, eliminate body odor, soothe inflammation, and improve the respiratory system.

Eucalyptus

Eucalyptus essential oil helps treat respiratory problems, muscle pains, fever, diabetes, and mental exhaustion. It is also a great help in skin and dental care.

Frankincense

Frankincense essential oil is best for wounds, infections, scars, digestion, coughs, and colds. It can also help uplift the mood, soothe anxiety, and promote cell regeneration.

Geranium

Geranium essential oil stops hemorrhaging, heals scars, tones the body, kills parasites, eliminates body odor, and promotes cell regeneration.

Ginger

Ginger essential oil is famous for curing pain, protecting the skin, inhibiting bacterial growth, improving memory, expelling phlegm, improving stomach health, and removing toxins.

Grapefruit

This essential oil can stimulate urination, prevent infection, reduce symptoms of depression, uplift mood, and eliminate toxins.

Helichrysum

This essential oil fights allergies, prevent microbial growth, reduces spasms and inflammations, heals scars and wounds, stimulates correct bile discharge, and helps regenerate cells.

Hyssop

Hotspot essential oil induces the tightening of skin, gums, and muscles. It helps eliminate excess gas, reduce spasms, promote healthy digestion, and increase urination and sweating.

Jasmine

Jasmine essential oil fights depression, removes the blues, cures sexual dysfunction, increases libido, regulates menstrual flow, increases milk production, eases labor pains, and relieves coughs and phlegm.

Juniper

Juniper essential oil protects wounds from infections, increases urination and sweating, brings radiance to the skin, purifies blood, cures rheumatism, reduces gas, and speeds up the healing of cuts.

Lavender

Lavender essential oil deals effectively with the nervous system, respiratory system, flow of urine, immune system, insomnia, and skin.

Book 7:
Native American Spirituality

Chapter 1: Native Americans Beliefs And Practices
Understanding Native American Beliefs And Practices

Native American beliefs and practices are one of the most fascinating aspects of the culture. With so much history and meaning behind them, it's no wonder that they have retained a large presence in modern-day society. This section will explore some of the most common Native American beliefs and practices. From animal symbolism to health practices, you will be enlightened on everything you need to know about these fascinating ancient cultures.

Definition Of Native American Spirituality

Native American spirituality is rooted in the spiritual traditions of the indigenous peoples of North America. These traditions embody a deep connection to the natural world and reverence for ancestors and spirits. Native American spirituality includes animism, Diné bizaad, and ikéyátsoyii. Animism holds that all things have a soul, including inanimate objects. Diné bizaad refers to the belief that everyday objects and natural phenomena have a spirit or power. ikéyátsoyii means "the way of the heart." This term refers to the idea that something within each person allows them to connect with their spiritual Source. Native Americans use ceremonies and rituals to commune with their spiritual Selves and honor their ancestors. They also rely on sweat lodges, dream questing, and other practices to access wisdom and knowledge about life, the universe, and human nature.

Spiritual Practice And Beliefs

They Don't Have Any Distinction Between the Spiritual And Physical World

Native American spirituality revolves around the connection between the spiritual and physical world. They don't have any distinction between the spiritual and physical world. Everything is connected, and everything has a spirit.

The tribes believe that the spirits of all things are alive and active. This includes plants, animals, and even inanimate objects. The Sioux say that everything in the world has a spirit and that it is important to respect these spirits.

Tribes also believe that there are many different types of spirits. Some are good, while others are evil. It is important to stay out of the way of these evil spirits, as they can cause great harm to people and their homes.

Native Americans Have Vast Religious Diversity

Native Americans have diverse religious beliefs and practices, some of which are linked to their ancestral spiritual traditions. Many Native Americans believe in a pantheon of powerful spiritual beings, including the creator god, the thunder god, the moon goddess, and other nature spirits. Some tribes practice animism, believing that all living things have a soul. Other tribes follow shamanic rituals and use traditional medicines and ceremonies to seek spiritual guidance.

Understanding Their Beliefs Related To Death

Native American beliefs about death are different from most people's. For the indigenous people of North America, death is not a finality. Instead, it is seen as transitioning into another world or state of being.

People indigenous to North America often believe that after someone dies, they go through four stages: the journey to the dead person's world or spirit village, the meeting with important spirits, the trial by ghost warriors, and finally, entering the eternal world. During each stage of their journey, natives undergo various trials and tribulations to prove themselves worthy of entering the eternal world.

Some beliefs suggest that during our earthly life, we are visited by various relatives and friends who have died. These visits help us learn some of the lessons we need to learn to move on to our final destination.

Another belief is that when someone dies, their spirit can still be seen and interacted with by those close to them. This means that if someone you love dies suddenly, it's not necessarily goodbye – you may still be able to communicate with them through mediums such as dreams or visions.

It is also common for native people to believe in reincarnation. After someone dies, their spirit may enter another body to continue living on earth. In fact, many cultures believe that every human being has been born at least once before – this is known as pre-birth incarnation. As we grow older and experience pain and suffering on earth, some of these experiences may help us prepare for our next life.

Festivals For Harvesting Or Planting

Fresh-picked produce is a popular tradition for many people worldwide, but what about Native Americans? Here are five festivals that celebrate the harvest or planting season.

1. The Navajo Harvest Festival takes place in September and celebrates the bounty of the year's crops. This festival features traditional dances, ceremonies, and singalongs.
2. The Cherokee Oktoberfest takes place in October and celebrates Germany's heritage on Cherokee land. Local beer, food, and music are all featured attractions of this event.
3. The Hmong New Year Festival is held in November to commemorate the end of the agricultural cycle and to pray for good crops for the coming year. There are many festivities, including a parade, cultural performances, and a fireworks show at nightfall.
4. The Hawaiian Festival of Aunty Lilo takes place in December to honor lady plants and fertility spirits associated with agriculture and hula dancing. Various festivals are held throughout the island chain throughout December, such as pig races, luau dances, marching band concerts, firework displays, etc.
5. The Pilipino Harvest Festival is celebrated in October in San Francisco, where Filipino immigrants live and work. This festival features colorful floats depicting scenes from traditional Filipino culture, food booths selling Sinigang (a type of soup made from fermented pork blood), games like karaoke and Pinoy Pong (a board game similar to checkers), as well as a nightly fireworks display.

Native American Ceremony Of The Pipes

No one knows when or where the ceremonial usage of pipes began, but it is considered very ancient. There are many different stories and myths surrounding using pipes, but one common belief is that they were used to communicate with spirit beings. Some believe the pipes were also used as musical instruments to summon spirits.

The modern ceremony of the pipe is a sacred time for Native Americans. It is an opportunity to connect with nature and the heavens. Each ceremony has unique elements, but most involve ceremonial smoke sticks and drums. The smoke from the pipe allows participants to commune with their ancestors and other spiritual beings.

Smudging

Smudging is a traditional ceremony practiced by many Native American tribes. It cleanses and purifies areas or objects and communicates with the natural world's spirits.

There are many different types of smudging ceremonies, but they all share some common elements. First, participants gather together around an object or area that needs cleansing. They then take some kind of burning material, such as sage, cedar wood, or sweetgrass, and light it on fire. The fire's heat helps release the plants' fragrances into the air. These scents are said to appeal to the spirits of nature, who can help to clean and protect the area or object being smudged.

After lighting the incense, participants often chant or sing prayers while waving their hands in front of the flame. This dancing and moving help distribute the smoke throughout the room and across the object or area being cleansed.

Sometimes people will massage oils (like lavender) over their bodies while performing this ritual to promote relaxation and ease stress.

Smudging is often used in traditional ceremonies like sweat lodges and dream quests. By working together, these rituals help to build connections between people and nature – a vital part of Native American culture.

Quests For Vision

Vision quests are a common practice in many Native American cultures. They are usually undertaken by young men to gain spiritual knowledge and power. A Vision quest typically involves a series of challenges the participant must complete gaining insight into his or her identity and purpose in life. These challenges can take many forms, including walking alone through difficult terrain, fasting, and prolonged prayer sessions. A vision quest's goal is to gain spiritual insight, physical strength, and stamina, which can be used later in life.

Death-Related Beliefs

In general, Native American religion followed the same trajectory as most other civilizations across the globe regarding death. They trust in a spirit that continues to exist after the physical body has died.

It will go to another world or spirit world, where it will have a similar life while in a human body on Earth. Considering that several tribes initially spent so much time traveling, the notion of traveling to another realm makes sense. They might see a voyage as a natural part of life. However, in certain instances, the spirit remains trapped on Earth or does not reach the spirit world.

Funeral rituals and ceremonies were established to aid the spirit's transition to the next life. This, however, is not all that unlike other faiths across the globe. Ancient Egyptian pharaohs, for example, were mummified & buried with worldly goods so that they might "live" happily after death. In Catholicism, "Last Rites" and prayers during a funeral offer the same functions.

Sweat Lodges

Sweat lodges have been around for centuries, dating back to when Native Americans pursued a kind of physical L spiritual purification and vision questing. Sweat lodges, also known as purification lodges, are places where you may refresh yourself and establish an unbreakable connection with the spiritual realm. Different tribes use different ways to achieve this objective, but it begins with a tiny wooden frame, sheets or skins to cover it, and a heat source. Spiritual leaders in the congregation arrange and choreograph them, giving particular instructions depending on the individual situation or objectives.

Offerings, prayers, and different kinds of tobacco, cedar, & sweetgrass to burn are all part of every sweat lodge ritual. Outside the lodge, a fire is constructed to heat rocks, which would then be brought inside for the duration. Water is placed on the rocks to release the aromatic and possibly mind-altering steam. Separately or in a group, they may be completed.

Ceremony of the Pipes

In Native American rituals, smoke & steam in different forms plays an important part. It represented a link between the ground below and the heavens above since it soared in the air. Anybody who has watched an old "Cowboys and Indians" movie or animation has most likely seen American Indians burning a peace pipe as a kind of ritual. These are implausible and oversimplified illustrations of the spiritual significance of pipe rituals.

Tobacco is also frequently utilized in spiritual ceremonies and rituals. During these rituals, several tribes pass around or smoke various pipes in the cardinal directions. The rituals are as varied as the tribes that carry them out and the circumstances they are carried out. Peace talks, naming rituals, and personal prayers all include pipe smoking. The pipe is supplied by a professional Pipe Carrier who coordinates the prayer process during multi-person events.

Chapter 2: Native Americans Spirituality In Medicines

Native Americans have healing practices that date back thousands of years. Many tribes had ways of combining roots, herbs, and other plant parts to heal their people. However, this does not imply that just herbs were employed in the Native American healing process.

No healing technique is the same when you travel from tribe to tribe. Still, you will see many parallels in their ceremonies, wisdom, and rituals. There were no therapeutic standards, but health was a manifestation of the spirit of Native Americans. They felt that no one would survive unless they healed the spirit, mind, and body. They needed to remain in their natural surroundings to avoid illness and injury. Of course, they realized they needed to heal their bodily issues to get healthier.

The herbal cures that came with these therapeutic methods were their main element, and they went beyond the aches and pains of the body. Of course, while they focused on the physical condition, they also informed the patient that focusing on their spirituality and internal harmony was necessary, providing many Native Americans the desire to survive numerous afflictions.

Many of the herbs used are still known today, as are many of the purposes they served. That doesn't mean that everything is as obvious as it was years ago when it was passed down from one person to the next.

Native American Medicine, as we know it today, refers to health techniques practiced by the many indigenous tribes who lived in America and Canada before the arrival of Europeans. The beliefs and practices differed per tribe, but there was a general idea that for there to be balance, there had to be harmony between the individual, the patient's family, the community, and the natural environment and that health and wellness depended on this.

Native American Medicine may be over 40,000 years old. Yet, most of it was not documented and was kept secret among many tribes until Europeans came 500 years ago. Most Native American elders are reluctant to share medical information for fear of losing or compromising holy knowledge. Some tribes, such as the Cherokee, recorded some medical knowledge. Still, the majority was passed down from generation to generation without being written down.

Many healers perished with this medicinal knowledge before Europeans could document some of it through observation. Native American tribes from the past and today are concerned with preserving their culture, and many healers are eager to learn about traditions and how they treat certain conditions. Although some elders believe that sharing health information with those outside their tribes will help preserve it, most do not trust sharing these secrets and remedies with non-natives. Therefore much remains undiscovered.

Americans have been mentioned in the US Pharmacopoeia at some point, implying that they have been and continue to be used by pharmaceutical companies to manufacture modern-day medicines.

The Importance of Spirituality

Spirituality was vital in Native American healing, as it has been throughout human history in most regions of the world. Prayers, singing, and dance was used in rituals and ceremonies. This aspect of spirituality distinguishes mainstream Medicine from the Native American healing procedure. Traditional Medicine seeks to restore a person's physical state. In contrast, native healers felt that spirituality and the emotional well-being of the individual, family, and community were essential for healing.

The Medicine Wheel

Like the Sacred Pipe, the medicine wheel is an old Native American (and not exclusively) concept whose objective was to reconcile the various components of one reality to their oneness.

We are made up of various personalities that dwell in the same body. Within you, you have the kid, the nurturing mother, the wise, the hot-tempered teenager, the hunter, and many other personalities.

Each is a part of you, and you cannot be you without them. There will be parts of you that are upset with you for not giving them the right thought and attention in the past and parts of you that take the stage much too frequently.

It is critical that you may create a strong relationship with all of your parts over time, providing them the appropriate space to express themselves so that they are pleased and feel valued.

You want them to be your life partner, not to work against your interests because they are disgruntled or dissatisfied. This wholeness is critical for your activities in life.

It's amazing how much this ancient and intuitive Native American notion parallels Carl Gustav Jung's Analytic Psychology. The subconscious, according to Jung, was not a place where detached memories and complexes were "stored," but rather, to use a metaphor, a complicated bundle of numerous archetypal characters.

Each personality has its own set of wants and abilities, and it interacts with others and the conscious ego. Everyone's psychic dynamics are formed by the relationships and struggles between personalities and between each personality and the awareness.

This notion can easily explain self-sabotage and any psychological inversion activity.

Before Jung, Native Americans were well aware of this concept, and most of their religious rites were centered on the reconciliation of opposites into the oneness of yourself.

It may take some time each day for a few months, but the effects and improvement in your day-to-day life will be astounding:

Find a quiet place where you can be alone for ten minutes daily. To relax, take two or three deep breaths and sit comfortably.

Assume you're wandering through a meadow. The sky is clear and blue on this sunny, gorgeous day. When you cross the grass, you only hear the wind blowing and the grass rustling. It's just you.

After some while, you come across an old home in the middle of the fields. When you open the front entrance, you are greeted by a large room with a large circular table in the center.

There are seats at the table. Many are taken by other humans or animals, while others are not. This is your personal circle.

Look for a comfortable chair. Take a seat and introduce yourself to everyone else present.

Who exactly are they? What is their backstory? What do they desire? How can you assist them?

Make an effort to get an agreement with all of your personas. You'll be astonished at how quickly your life will improve if you stop sabotaging yourself and acting selfishly.

The medicine wheel reflects this concept: we are a wholeness of several parts. We must find a way to live in good relationships with all of them to thrive in this life with balance and harmony.

This concept can be expanded from your own oneness to the oneness of your family, community, and so on to the entire cosmos.

Native Americans understood the simple truth of the many that are one. They developed the medicine wheel ceremonial to restore life's wholeness.

The practitioner must construct a stone circle for this ceremony. This simple act generates an upward spiral of good energy, and all the forces of life join to create this hallowed realm of unity and harmony.

By establishing a space of harmony and tranquility for himself, the practitioner returns some of the order and harmony he received to the Creator.

Each stone represents a community member or a part of your personality who is free to come and say whatever he or she wants.

The largest stone in the Circle signifies the Spirit, the core of everything, and is located in the Circle's heart.

The Circle of Stones includes four gates in each of the four directions (North, South, East, and West), each representing a different archetype:

South: Symbolizes the beginning, childhood, spring, hope, and vigor. It represents rebirth.

West: Adolescence, struggle, and the search for purpose and identity. It depicts our journeys into the darkest aspects of our personalities, our journey "into the shadow," as Jung put it, to discover who we truly are. We are deprived of the things we consider significant in this circle section. The West is a symbol of the agonizing breakdown.

North: This is the age of middle-age equilibrium, caring for others, and altruism.

It is the time of old age, rest, wisdom, and enlightenment in the East. It is the stage at which you renounce the entire material world and become more sensitive to the spiritual.

There is more beneath the surface of the sacred pipe and the medicine wheel. Each element has a deeper meaning and purpose and may be utilized to improve people's well-being.

Medicine of Native Americans Today

Because of the widespread concern about the side effects, toxicity, resistance, and addiction produced by pharmaceutical pharmaceuticals, surgery, and other contemporary treatments, there has been a boom in interest in Native American Medicine. People are looking for herbal treatments to help cure ailments and disorders. Quality herbal medicines have been developed over the years, most of which have been drawn from Native American medical traditions to heal medical ailments. Herbal medicines are effective, with fewer side effects and lower toxicity than pharmaceutical products.

You must select herbal treatments that have been produced with standard pharmaceutical materials.

While Native American Medicine was prohibited, many of the medications available today can be traced back to it. Laurance Johnston examined various treatment systems from throughout the world and discovered that many of the herbal remedies utilized by Native Americans are included in the United States Pharmacopoeia.

Native Americans, for example, employed the bark of the willow tree to cure pain. Acetylsalicylic acid was found in this bark. Aspirin is another name for acetylsalicylic acid.

There are, however, some significant philosophical contrasts between modern Medicine and Native American Medicine.

Book 8:
Native American Natural Medicine

Chapter 1: The Cherokee Legend

The Cherokee legend is one of Americana's most captivating and spellbinding tales. Spanning centuries, it tells the story of a people who faced many challenges—from war to disease to persecution to displacement. Here, we're going to explore this legend in-depth and provide you with everything you need to know so that you can understand it better. From its origins to its characters, this guide will take you on a journey through some of the most iconic Cherokee stories.

The Cherokee Legend: A Historical Overview

The Cherokee Legend is a deeply rooted story with a rich history. It has been passed down from generation to generation and remains a popular topic of discussion today. The legend tells the tale of two brothers, Coyote and Trapper, who were exiled from their tribe for breaking tribal laws. They journeyed through the world searching for a new home but never found peace. After years of wandering, they built their own homes in the sky.

While building their home, Coyote and Trapper encountered many challenges. First, they had to overcome the dangers of the wild world below. Second, they had to contend with the obstacles posed by their fellow tribespeople. Finally, they had to fight against nature to build their cabin high in the mountains. In the end, though, Coyote and Trapper founded their own tribe.

The Cherokee Legend is full of symbolism that speaks to the human experience. For example, Coyote and Trapper represent courage and determination; they can overcome all odds despite being outsiders. The tree that helps them reach their home represents growth and transformation; it is always there to help those willing to take advantage of its resources.

The Cherokee Legend is an inspiring story that celebrates perseverance and self-reliance. It teaches us that no matter what life throws our way, we can always find a way to triumph over adversity.

The Moccasin Maker: How the Cherokee Created an Epic Legend

The legend of the Cherokee moccasin maker is an epic story steeped in history and culture. The moccasin maker is a mythical character who is said to have created the first moccasins.

The legend starts with a woman named Mother Earth. She was angry because humans were littering her land and destroying everything she had created. So, she cursed humans with bad weather, poor health, and hard lives.

One day, a man named Thunderer went hunting in the forest. He came across a deer caught in a trap set by humans. The man could free the deer and kill the hunter who had set the trap. In honor of his deed, Thunderer became known as the great hunter-warrior who saved humanity from Mother Earth's wrath.

While he was hunting, Thunderer met a beautiful woman named Sky Woman. Sky Woman told him about Mother Earth's rage and how humans were responsible. She offered to help him save humanity if he married her. Thunderer agreed, and they got married soon after.

Together, they traveled to Mother Earth's home place to plead for forgiveness on behalf of humanity. After hearing their story, Mother Earth relented and permitted them to live on her land, provided they did not damage it or violate any of her rules.

Sky Woman started making moccasins for people to wear so they would not hurt their feet walking on the earth's surface. She also taught them how to cultivate crops and build homes.

Humans had learned their lesson, but they still did not live in harmony with Mother Earth. Thunderer and Sky Woman created a new legend telling of a great moccasin maker who would teach them how to live in harmony with nature.

This legendary figure was known as the formulate make. He or she was said to have created the first moccasins from the skins of animals that had died of natural causes. The formulate make also taught people how to weave baskets and make other items from natural materials.

The legend of the Cherokee moccasin maker is an epic story steeped in history and culture. The moccasin maker is a mythical character who is said to have created the first moccasins.

The Vision Quest: The Journey that Changed the Cherokee Nation Forever

The Cherokee Nation is one of North America's most picturesque, culturally rich, and historically significant tribes. Their land, known as "Cherokee Country," stretches from the Appalachian Mountains to the Gulf of Mexico. The tribe's long and revered history includes a unique vision quest ceremony known as the " Path of the Arrow."

The Path of the Arrow is an initiation rite that marks the transition from boyhood to manhood for Cherokee men. It involves a journey into nature and challenges participants to endure physical hardships to gain spiritual enlightenment. The journey leads them away from civilization and into the depths of the wilderness, where they must face fear, solitude, and self-discovery.

The Path of the Arrow has played an important role in shaping Cherokee culture. It has served as an inspiration to generations of Cherokees. They have followed in its footsteps and embraced their cultural heritage. Today, it remains an important symbol of identity for the tribe. It is seen as an integral part of their traditions and history.

The Battle of Horseshoe Bend: A Turning Point in the Cherokees' Struggle for Independence

The Battle of Horseshoe Bend is often considered a turning point in the Cherokee struggle for independence. The battle was fought on September 14, 1814, near the present-day town of Horseshoe Bend, Arkansas. After defeating the United States Army at the Battle of Tippecanoe in 1811, the Creek and Cherokee tribes were emboldened and believed they could defeat American troops again. However, at Horseshoe Bend, General Andrew Jackson led a tactical surprise attack against a smaller force of Cherokees unprepared for an assault. The victory resulted in a string of military successes that helped to unite the American colonies and eventually resulted in the War of 1812.

After the Revolution: The Legacy of the Cherokee Nation

The Cherokee Nation is one of the oldest nations in North America. After years of struggle, the nation could maintain its independence and sovereignty after the American Revolution.

Today, the Cherokee Nation enjoys a rich cultural heritage passed down from generation to generation. The nation's traditional values include strong family bonds, a deep reverence for nature, and a commitment to democracy.

The legacy of the Cherokee Nation will continue to be celebrated long after its people have passed away. Thanks to their efforts, the Cherokee Nation remains an important part of American history and culture.

Chapter 2: Sacred Medicines For Native Americans

Sacred Medicine is a centuries-old approach to Medicine rooted in indigenous Native American culture. Sacred Medicine is experiencing a renaissance, expanding and incorporating modern medicine ideas.

Sacred Medicine is a state of mind rather than a technique. You need to know this to get a better understanding of it.

What Exactly Is Sacred Medicine?

Many people identify Medicine with chilly, sterile facilities, medications, surgical procedures, and people dressed in white coats striving to improve a person's physical condition. On the other hand, Medicine was a complicated, interconnected spiritual and physical well-being process in ancient cultures, particularly among Native Americans.

Our bodies are separated into several elements: physical, mental, social, and spiritual. We feel sick and unwell when these factors are out of balance.

The indigenous people saw Medicine as a way to create balance and harmony with nature's basic powers. It meant being conscious of our power, which enables us to live in the world as a whole and complete people.

Because the indigenous people did not practice any Abrahamic religions, their lives were not based on interpretations or prohibitions issued by Holy Scriptures. Instead, they went to nature for answers, examining the world they lived in and studying its natural rhythms to teach us how to justify our position.

They believe that life does not exist in a straight line, as we measure it in terms of time and days, but rather in cycles or circles, similar to the phases of the sun and moon, seasons, and the circle of life. Our lives, as well as the lives of animals, plants, and herbs, are all part of a cycle.

With this awareness of existence, Sacred Medicine was born. It contains a sacred circle with medicinal characteristics that can heal our bodies, brains, and souls.

Indigenous Culture's Four Sacred Medicines

The Native Americans believe that the four Sacred Medicines that comprise the medical wheel are made up of four natural plants.

The medicinal wheel has four distinct characteristics because it operates in four directions. The center of the wheel, which represents the essence of the global one or divine essence, cannot be described. It's generally known as the "holy secret" in Native American culture.

The four directions of the wheel are defined differently by different tribes. They believe that each direction corresponds to different aspects of life. Hence it has diverse meanings for different tribes.

The wheel is divided into many colors, such as red, yellow, black, and white, each with its own meaning.

The following are some representations of the medical wheel:

It portrays life stages such as birth, adolescence, adulthood, and death. It also signifies the four seasons: spring, summer, winter, and fall. It can also reflect people's emotional, spiritual, intellectual, and physical characteristics. It also depicts natural elements such as air, fire, water, and earth. Some believe the various directions reflect human races, such as black, white, Asian, and American Indian. It can also represent creatures like the eagle, bear, buffalo, and wolf (Sol, 2021).

The Four Sacred Medicines are the most essential representations of the medicine wheel.

Tobacco was the first plant ever given to indigenous peoples by the Creator. They think it is the first plant spirit to ignite all others. Other plants considered sacred Medicine include sage, cedar, and sweet grass. All of these plants are regarded as the four Sacred Medicines.

These Sacred Medicines are used by Native Americans in their daily lives and ceremonies. All these plants are used for smudging; white sage, cedar, and sweet grass have various applications. The indigenous people think that each plant represents a different entryway. Tobacco leads to the eastern door, while sage leads to the western door. The Southern door is occupied by sweet grass, while the Northern door is occupied by cedar. When burned, the pleasant perfume of the smoke produced by these sacred plants is intended to placate the spirits they revere and praise (Ojibwe Journal, n.d.).

Movement For Modern Sacred Medicine

The current Sacred Medicine movement is founded on old concepts but with some modern twists. This movement's adherents characterize it as collaborating with the mind, body, and spirit. It emphasizes the heart, places a premium on intuition and seeks to empower its adherents. It also believes in a more feminine approach to healing. This gentler approach encompasses physical and mental health and other elements of our existence. These include variables that many doctors overlook, such as our professional well-being, financial health, spiritual well-being, the effectiveness of our environment, and our ability to maintain interpersonal relationships.

These factors have a long-term impact on our bodies health, and modern Sacred Medicine tries to treat all of these issues concurrently.

The current Sacred Medicine movement advocates that if the body's parts are balanced, it may heal itself. This is not to dismiss the benefits of contemporary Medicine. It entails blending the best of what modern Medicine offers with traditional beliefs. Our bodies are magnificent; we all have the incredible ability to heal ourselves; we simply need to know how to activate it.

This movement seeks to lessen our reliance on chemical Medicine. Practitioners of modern Sacred Medicine hope to empower their patients to tap into their healing intuition and initiate their healing process.

Modern Sacred Medicine practitioners value their participation in the healing process just as much as doctors do. Nobody knows our bodies like we do. Based on our intuition about how to treat us, we can assist our doctors in developing beneficial remedies.

Sacred Medicine is a growing movement among both healthcare providers and patients. What is the movement's goal? Its goal is to "reclaim medicine's, lost heart." They feel that Medicine has devolved into a cold and uncaring profession, and they want to restore compassion and spirituality to the profession (Rankin, n.d.b).

Sacred Medicine practitioners believe strongly in the healing power of love. They acknowledge that science can treat symptoms, but they think true healing results from love. Following Sacred Medicine does not imply dismissing the healing abilities of contemporary Medicine, surgery, or any other kind of treatment. Rather, it suggests that simply treating a symptom or removing an organ does not constitute recovery. Modern Sacred Medicine believes that to properly recover, you must address the source of the problem. Only you know the state of your heart; you must identify the source of your problem, determine why you are experiencing discomfort, and attempt to resolve it from the inside (Rankin, n.d.a).

Sacred Medicine In Everyday Life

Some modern Sacred Medicine principles can be implemented in our daily lives. These are their names:

1. We can use illnesses, injuries, and trauma as opportunities for spiritual awakening, especially if we are willing to accept our suffering as a necessary part of our progress.
2. Our bodies have the potential to heal themselves. Still, chronic stress reduces our ability to heal, compromising the body's natural functioning.
3. This covers your relationships, profession, sexuality, spirituality, income, food, and physical movements.
4. Working out, eating right, getting enough sleep, and taking your medication is the minimum; they will not lead you to peak levels of wellness and health.
5. You claim to desire to get cured, but your inner saboteur interferes with the healing process.
6. You, not anybody else, are the expert on your body.
7. Have faith in the healing power of love.
8. Have faith in the power of circles.
1. When your life force is depleted, you can absorb it from others.

2. 11. Use your energy and life force to heal others; you can also cure yourself this way.
3. 12. You must generate your life energy to be at the peak of your health.
4. 13. Strong relationships can act as powerful forces for healing.
5. 14. You require a safe haven, a sanctuary, to heal.
6. 15. Don't be scared to laugh and have fun; it's the finest therapy.

Chapter 3: Main Native Americans Medicinal Plants

Growing medicinal herbs and plants at home is a requirement for every herb garden lover serious about their hobby. If you like gardening, the apothecary mentality of medicinal plants may be a natural step for you into medicine! Create a delightful herb garden that also serves as a source of beneficial health supplements. You can produce wonderful anti-inflammatory and immunity-boosting ointments and drinks with high-quality herbs. If you have a little information, you and your family will be on the road to improved health. You can easily grow medicinal herbs in your home, garden, pots, and even in tight spaces.

Basil

Growing basil is simple and adaptable enough to flourish both inside and outdoors. It can convert everyday dishes into gourmet marvels! Unlike dried basil, fresh basil has a distinct flavor and texture. In addition to flatulence, basil is a medicinal plant that may assist with a lack of appetite, wounds, scrapes, and other minor ailments (intestinal gas).

Types of basil to plant at home

- Cinnamon basil smells like sweet spice and has unusually beautiful and fragrant flowers.
- Lemon basil includes Citral, an aromatic chemical in citrus fruits that gives it a distinct lemony flavor and scent.
- Purple basil is often planted for its ornamental qualities, as well as for its fragrance and blossoms.
- It's possible to grow perennial basils that come back year after year, such as African Blue basil, which has beautiful blue veins on its leaves, and Thai basil. Still, most other kinds are annuals that need replanted yearly.
- Globe and Greek basil are much more challenging to grow but form pretty little bushes that stay well-contained.
- To cultivate basil, start by sowing seeds four to six weeks before the final frost date of the calendar year. Basil requires warm air and sun-

light to thrive; therefore, starting the seeds inside rather than outside to avoid being harmed by frost is typically the most convenient option. Keep the soil damp but not soaked. Basil plants are happy with 6-8 hours of sunlight a day.

Cayenne

Cayenne - an excellent plant for your apothecary arsenal - is botanically not considered an herb. On the other hand, many people think cayenne peppers are the king of medicinal herbs. These peppers have been utilized for thousands of years to treat various health issues. The therapeutic effects of cayenne peppers are complemented by the fact that they are excellent for cooking and contain several healthy elements.

Cayenne peppers may be found in many dishes. They are members of the nightshade family of flowering plants, including bell peppers and jalapenos, and are closely related to them. Christopher Columbus introduced them to Europe in the 15th century after discovering them in Central and South America and bringing them back to Europe.

In addition to being a popular spice used in many various regional forms of cooking, cayenne peppers have been utilized medicinally by early South American civilizations for hundreds of thousands of years. These peppers have an outstanding nutritional profile, containing a wide range of antioxidants that are good for your overall health and well-being.

This is due to the active chemical in cayenne peppers, capsaicin, which is responsible for the peppers' therapeutic effects. It also contributes to their spicy flavor. The amount of capsaicin in a dash of cayenne pepper determines how hot it is. The amount of capsaicin present determines how hot it is. The science-backed benefits of cayenne pepper include metabolism-boosting properties, reduced production of the hunger hormone ghrelin, lowering of blood pressure, aiding digestion through the delivery of enzymes to the stomach, and pain-relieving properties through the reduction of the amount of substance.

Chamomile

Chamomile is a flowering plant that produces delicate, daisy-like blooms. These blooms may be dried and used to produce herbal teas that are both calming and therapeutic, as well as hot compresses and infused oils for skincare. The cultivation of this charming and useful small herb in your yard is not difficult at all. Seeds may be started either inside or outdoors. After that, you'll need to take good care of your chamomile plants until the blooms are ready to be harvested. These plants enjoy a sunny spot and regular watering.

Chamomile is known for its apple scent. It helps immensely to help heal the skin, reduce any dryness and itchiness, and reduce inflammation in irritated skin. The herb also helps immensely when relieving indigestion, tension, anxiety, and tension.

Lavender

Lavender is one of the herbs which offer medicinal properties by just breathing it. While most herbs work when you consume them, lavender works even when someone has just decided to smell it. When breathed, the herb has a soothing and relaxing effect, which is one of the key reasons people use it in baths, hospitals, and their beds to rest. If you're interested in aromatherapy, lavender is the most important element. Most people who get such services are treated to rooms, towels, and basically all clothes soaked in lavender. For physical uses, lavender is used in treating burns and abrasions.

Light for at least 8 hours every day.

Sage

The word sage is derived from its genus, "salvia," which means, " to heal." Currently, sage is used as both a herb and a spice. In the early days, the herb was just looked upon for its medicinal properties, and rarely did it gain recognition as a delicacy. Studies show that the continued use of sage helps fight sore throats, memory issues, blood cholesterol issues, and mood swings.

Savory and somewhat bitter, sage (Salvia officinalis) is a hardy perennial (growing in zones 5 to 9) with a fragrant flavor. Sage thrives in a wide range of climates and can withstand temperatures as low as 0 degrees Fahrenheit (32 degrees Celsius). It has a lovely appearance in the garden and blooms with beautiful purple, pink, blue, or white flowers throughout the summer months. Only water sage plants when the soil is dry to the touch.

Easy to grow and easy to appreciate, lavender (Lavandula) is a welcome addition to any garden, with its beautiful flowers and a pleasant aroma. Lavender is a Mediterranean herb that thrives in hot, sunny locations. Identify a location in your garden where the plant will get direct sun.

Lemon Balm

Growing Lemon Balm at home provides various options, from healing minor wounds and skin disorders to relieving pain and swelling of insect bites. Mosquitoes, in particular, stay away from Lemon Balm. It can also treat cold sores, soothe sore muscles, and regulate blood sugar.

Rosemary

Rosemary is an excellent choice for a rock garden or planting at the top of a dry stone wall. The plant may be cultivated as a perennial shrub in Zones 7 and higher temperatures. If you live in a colder climate, it should be grown in pots and brought inside during the winter. Water when the soil feels dry and re-pot as the plant get bigger and the roots fill the pot. Rosemary enjoys 6-8 hours of direct sunlight.

Thyme

Thyme is evergreen and a member of the mint family Lamiaceae; it is a wonderfully versatile plant. It does best in full sun. Ensure that Thyme is planted in well-drained soil with a pH of about 7.0, and you can also add limestone, oyster shells, or crushed eggshell to plants when planting.

Parsley

Historically and today, parsley is heralded for its nutritional value: Flavinoids, antioxidants that neutralize free radicals. Some of these have been shown to prevent (or slow) the development of certain cancers. Parsley also has many rich vitamins, including vitamins L, 812, K, and A. Parsley helps keep your immune system healthy, heals the nervous system, and tones your bones.

Parsley is slow to germinate, so if you begin with seeds, do this in the Spring, eight weeks indoors before the last freeze. Also, soak seeds for 24 hours in warm water before planting, which will speed up germination. Beginning by seed in the Spring will give the plant plenty of time to acclimate before Fall arrives and the first frost hits. Plant in full or partial sun; it will thrive in both conditions. A loamy soil fertilized with natural ingredients is required for an excellent growing result.

If you suffer from mental health disorders like depression, I highly recommend considering St. John's wort. The plant has several active parts, including the leaves and its yellow flowers. However, care must be taken since this herb is also associated with some elements of harm and danger. This herb, coupled with other medicinal herbs, seemingly reacts whenever mixed up with other medications, particularly contemporary ones. Therefore, if you are trying to solve any mental problem, you must desist from mixing it with any other medicines and technically take it on its own.

There are certain seasons where the herb is highly prevalent, including mid-summer until Fall. The significant benefit of this herb is that it is straightforward to adapt to different environmental conditions and thus can grow in literally any locality under perfect circumstances. The herb can be found in the driest places, such as where you typically find cacti, and most people marvel at its tenacity.

Marigold

Marigold is a herb that may be beneficial for various skin conditions, including sunburn, acne, blemishes, ulcers, and stomach disorders. Marigold, also known as Calendula, is one of the most effective all-purpose skin treatments. It is especially effective for small wounds, burns, bug bites, dry skin, and acne. Acne may be treated with calendula tea used topically twice or thrice daily as an astringent face rinse. Many remedies, such as salves, creams, and lotions, are accessible over-the-counter (OTC).

Even though marigolds are quite simple to cultivate, they are available in a wide range of hues. These include white, yellow, orange, red, and mixed colors. Marigolds are also available in various sizes, ranging from miniatures less than a foot tall to huge kinds that may reach up to four feet. Even though marigolds are tough plants, they are susceptible to death in cold temperatures.

Marigolds thrive in full light and normal garden soil and are quite simple to cultivate from seed. It's also possible to grow them in pots or containers, which is why they're referred to as "pot marigolds." The sticky blossoms of the calendula plant must be harvested every two to three days to guarantee a longer blossoming season. Unless you thoroughly mulch the Calendula, it will normally self-seed. It is normally grown annually, but it may also be a short-lived perennial in warmer climates.

Book 9:
Native American Stones & Crystals

Chapter 1: Basic Things To Know About Healing Stones And Crystals

Healing Crystals are probably one of the most popular topics in the world today. Whether you're a skeptic or believer, there's no denying that these stones have powerful effects on our physical and emotional health. This guide will provide you with an overview of what healing crystals are, how to use them, and what their benefits are. We also have a few recommendations for some of the best healing crystals for various issues. So dive in and learn everything you need to know about healing crystals.

Given our current love for crystals and their therapeutic potential, it's amazing (and disheartening) to consider how frequently communities with deep links with stones have been attacked by colonizers and explorers for their "barbaric" and "uneducated" practices.

Though more harsh fronts had been made for generations earlier, the "Code of Indian Offenses" threatened the customary position of medicine men and women in indigenous society in the late nineteenth century. If they are barred from utilizing healing equipment such as crystals, these healers may face prison or worse.

Native American gemstones in traditional, ceremonial use have a rich history that includes perspectives from over 2,000 unique tribes of indigenous people in North America alone.

While we cannot cover all of the meanings and applications of crystals in Native American healing practices, we hope to raise awareness of this important diversity and provide a glimpse into the vast array of holy crystal connections.

Healing Stones' Importance in Native American Culture

Native American gemstones are important in healing individuals and uniting indigenous societies as tools and totems. In indigenous cultures, health symbolizes spiritual life and ongoing efforts to strengthen it and keep the physical body in harmony with nature.

Personal Treatment with Healing Stones

Many indigenous people believe that illness and harm occur when a person loses touch with and harmony with the natural world and that health is balanced with the natural world. Discord is caused by a person's thoughts and behaviors. A person with negative habits, poor thoughts, or unpleasant emotions invites the consequences of an imbalance with nature's perfect, positive gifts.

A person can seek treatment from a medicine man or woman in these natural healing traditions. Medicine men and women provided therapy in indigenous communities using alternative healing practices such as crystals and holy symbols. As previously said, crystal connections are very subtle and unique to each individual. Individual therapeutic methods in indigenous healing traditions reveal this relationship.

Healing with sacred items such as crystals and other spiritual rituals is a very intimate and private experience shared between the healer and the patient. The patient's preferences take precedence in terms of how to approach and incorporate different methods into treatment.

Before healing with crystals or other talismans, the medicine person respects and listens to the individual's vibrations.

Healing Stones for Social Harmony

An individual's illness profoundly influences a tribe's close-knit group. As a result, medicine men and women are also concerned with community healing.

They assist the community in understanding how one person's disharmony throws the entire community out of balance with nature. The negative energy that afflicts an individual might spread to the entire community. The community may suffer collectively due to communal decisions and behaviors rather than simply due to a single sick individual.

Traditional indigenous healers officiate over rites and ceremonies that remove the remaining energy of illness and weakness to reinvigorate the community and restore it to balance with nature, using Native American gemstones, potent symbols, and plants like sage or palo santo.

The extraordinary abilities that indigenous people developed to work with healing stones and crystals attest to the advanced methods that Native American tribes have used for ages.

Long lines of practice resulted in the skill to polish smooth crystals, carve stone features, and weave elaborate designs. As a result of these abilities, Native American healing stones found numerous applications in their society.

Relationship with Spirit Guides

Native American gemstones make the connection between humans and spirit guides tangible. Certain stones are thought to summon spirits and invite them into human contact.

Native Americans build a natural, balanced protection with the Earth by storing crystals. They can also access various divine worlds using crystals and other sacred artifacts and substances, such as peyote.

Keeping a Historical Record

The design of crystal ornaments and jewelry worn as amulets tells long-held oral traditions and indigenous history stories. Symbols precisely engraved into crystals and gemstones contribute to preserving some aspects of Native American culture.

Economy and Trade

While the spiritual significance of crystals and stones for indigenous people has persisted over time, their craft of employing these materials in jewelry and other uses incorporated new patterns and production technology developed through trade.

These influences came about as a result of economic networks and people movement. Not all migration into these communities resulted in beneficial outcomes, such as the introduction of starvation and illness. However, indigenous people did find significant markets for their meticulously crafted crystal art.

What Are Crystals?

Crystals are naturally occurring substances that are made up of atoms that are arranged in a specific way. These substances can be solid, liquid, or gas. Crystals can be found in many different shapes and sizes and often have unique properties that make them useful for healing. Crystals can help improve physical and mental health, protect against radiation and other toxins, and promote positive energy. They can also help to connect people with the spiritual world.

To use crystals for healing, it is important to know what types of crystals are best suited for your specific needs. Some common crystals include quartz, jasper, turquoise, apatite, amethyst, peridot, chalcedony, calcite, rose quartz, and onyx. It is also helpful to know the properties of the crystal you are using. For example, quartz protects against radiation damage, while rose quartz is beneficial for improving emotional well-being.

What Are The Common Benefits Of Healing Crystals?

There are many benefits to using healing crystals for your health and well-being. These crystals have a long history of being used for healing purposes, and there is evidence to support their effectiveness. Here are some of the most common benefits of using healing crystals:

Healing Crystals Can Help Reduce Stress

Stress can cause several health problems, including high blood pressure, heart disease, and diabetes. Heating crystals can help reduce stress levels by balancing energy in the body. They can also help improve sleep quality and promote a more relaxed mood.

Healing Crystals Can Help Reduce Anxiety And Depression

Anxiety and depression are both major mental health issues that can be difficult to treat. Healing crystals may help by providing calming energy and promoting positive thinking. They can also help boost your immune system and relieve pain.

Healing Crystals Can Help Relieve Pain

Many people use healing crystals to relieve pain from physical conditions such as arthritis, back pain, or headaches. Heating crystals may work by balancing energy in the body, relieving inflammation, and stimulating the nerves that control pain sensations.

Healing Crystals Can Help Improve Mental Health

Many people use healing crystals to improve their mental health. They may provide energy and positive thinking, which can help reduce anxiety and depression. Crystals may also help boost your immune system and relieve pain.

How Should You Choose The Right Crystal For You?

There are many types of crystals to choose from when looking for a healing stone, but not all crystals work the same way. It's important to select the right crystal for your needs.

To decide what type of crystal is best for your situation, ask yourself these questions:

-What do I need to heal?

-What is my intention?

-Am I using this crystal as a supplemental aid or primary tool?

-How will I be using it?

Suppose you are trying to heal an ailment such as depression, anxiety, or grief. In that case, quartz is a good choice because it amplifies energy and can help clear blocks in the energetics. If you use this crystal as part of a ritual or meditation practice, then amethyst or tourmaline would be better because they promote peace and tranquility.

If you are only looking to calm your nerves or increase energy levels, then any variety of calcite or apatite would be appropriate. Remember that some crystals attract more negative energy than others, so it is important to experiment with different stones until you find what works best for you.

How Do Healing Crystals Work?

The power of crystals to heal comes from their unique structure and how they resonate with the universe's energy. Crystals are made up of molecules that are arranged in specific patterns and structures. This gives them the ability to store and release energy.

Crystals have been used for centuries as beauty, meditation, and healing objects. They are said to have various properties that can help us improve our well-being. Healing crystals can help us connect with our spiritual side and increase our awareness of our innermost energies.

When choosing a healing crystal, it is important to research its properties before using it. Different crystals can work better depending on their particular health issues or needs. It is also important to remember that not all crystals are suitable for everyone due to their sensitive nature. Before using a crystal for healing purposes, it is always recommended to test it on a small scale first to see if it is compatible with your energy body.

How To Use Your Crystal

There is no one answer to how to use crystals for healing. However, some basic guidelines can help you get started.

When using crystals for healing, it is important to know your energy level and the condition you are trying to heal. You should also keep in mind the qualities of the crystal you are using. For example, use a crystal with Heart energy properties if you are working on repairing a heart issue. If you are working on releasing anger or stress, use an Earth-based crystal such as turquoise or amethyst.

Once you have determined what kind of crystal you need, it is important to cleanse and charge it before using it for healing. To do this, place the crystal in a bowl of warm water and sprinkle it with rose petals or lavender buds. Allow the crystal to soak up the water, then rinse it well. Be sure to dry it off completely before using it.

Another key step in using crystals for healing is visualization. When thinking about what you want to heal, picture the health improvement accompanied by the visualized energy of the healer stone(s). This can help attune yourself more fully to your intended outcome while using crystals for healing.

How To Store Your Crystals Safely

When it comes to crystals, many people have a lot of questions. How do they work? What are their benefits? How can I use them for healing?

There are many ways to store crystals, and the best way for each person depends on their needs and preferences. Here are some tips for keeping your crystals safe:

-Store crystals in a dark, cool place away from direct sunlight or heat.

-Make sure the crystal container is airtight to keep out moisture and other elements.

-Do not leave crystal containers open to the air - they can attract dust and other elements that can damage the crystals.

-If you're going to travel with your crystals, make sure to pack them in a secure container and protect them from moisture and light.

Chapter 2: Most Used Crystals And Stones

Native Americans have used crystals and rocks for centuries to heal themselves and their surroundings. These natural resources have many benefits from soothing wounds to balancing energy within the body. Today, the popularity of crystals and rocks continues to grow as people seek natural remedies for various health problems. This section will explore some of the healing properties of crystals and rocks used by Native American shamans. By incorporating crystal healing into your own health regimen, you can achieve numerous benefits specific to your body chemistry. So read on, and learn about one of nature's most versatile healing tools!

Red Jasper

The red jasper is a popular healing crystal many Native American tribes use. It is believed to help clear the mind, promote concentration, and help with stress relief. The jasper is also considered protective and helpful in bringing good luck.

Quartz

Quartz crystals and rocks have been used by indigenous people for centuries to enhance their physical and spiritual well-being. The stones are said to help balance the energies in the body, clear energy blocks, amplify positive vibrations, and encourage positive thinking. Some of the most common healing properties attributed to quartz include enhancing energy flow and reducing stress, anxiety, depression, and other mental health issues.

Turquoise

Turquoise is the gemstone of choice for many Native American healers. The Aztec word for turquoise, chalchihuitl, means "turquoise stone." The Mayans used a blue variety of turquoise called "malachite" to color their pottery and tombs. Today, turquoise is still an important stone for Native Americans.

Some believe turquoise has spiritual properties because of its unique color and hardness. It is also thought to be beneficial in healing physical and emotional issues. Some tribes use it as a talisman against bad luck or disease. In contrast, others use it to enhance mental clarity and concentration.

The Cherokee believed that turquoise could help them see into the future and protect them from harm. Many people use it as a protective stone against negative energy and stress.

Granite

Granite is a type of rock found in many parts of the world. Native Americans have used granite for centuries to heal themselves and their communities. There are many reasons why granite is such a powerful healing stone.

Granite contains minerals such as feldspar, quartz, and mica. These minerals help to detoxify the body and support the immune system. Granite also has strong energy vibrations, which can help to clear emotional blockages and promote healing.

Native American tribes use different types of granite for different purposes. For example, the Navajo people use red granite to relieve stress and improve concentration. The Mohawk people use white granite to help them connect with their spirit guides and heal physical ailments.

Sandstone

Sandstone is a type of sedimentary rock that is composed of finely-grained minerals. This type of rock is often found near the Earth's surface and can be used to create jewelry ornaments, sculptures, or buildings. Native American people have long utilized sandstone to create tools and objects used for healing purposes.

Native Americans believe sandstone has special healing properties because it helps clear energy blockages and balances the chakras. Many people use sandstone to massage their temples and other parts of their bodies to promote good health and restore balance. Some people also use sandstone to cleanse negative energies from their homes or businesses.

Some people believe that sandstone's vibrations can help stimulate psychic abilities. In contrast, others believe it can help relieve stress or tension. In either case, using sandstone as part of a holistic approach toward wellness is believed to be beneficial for both the mind and body.

Azurite

Azurite is a colorful mineral that is found in many places around the world. It's often used to heal wounds because it helps stimulate the immune system. Native Americans use azurite to treat illnesses and injuries. They believe it has the power to remove negative energy from the body.

Black Onyx

Black Onyx is a type of quartz mostly found in Mexico and Peru. It is believed to have spiritual properties and is often used by Native Americans to heal wounds, clear energy blockages, and bring peace.

One of the main reasons Black Onyx is so popular among Native American healers is that it can absorb negative energy and transform it into positive energy. This makes it a perfect stone for clearing out any negative energies that may be causing you stress or physical pain.

Another major benefit of black onyx is that it can help to harmonize your chakras. Balancing your chakras can improve your overall well-being and connect with your spiritual pathway.

Tiger's Eye

Tiger's eye is a popular gemstone used by many native American tribes. It is said to have protective properties and has been used as an amulet for centuries. The color of the tiger's eye ranges from blue to black, with the most popular being a deep blue.

The stone is named after the tiger's sigil on the coats of arms of various European monarchies. The first recorded use of the name comes from a Greek work entitled 'On stones,' written in the 2nd century BC. In Asia, it was known as topaz. It was used by Alexander the Great and his army during their conquest of India in 327 BC.

There are many stories about how the gem became associated with certain powers or beliefs. One story tells that an Indian prince discovered the mineral while hunting and kept it hidden because he thought it would bring him great power. A princess who found it fell in love with him, but he refused to give it to her because he knew its true power could only be wielded by royalty. Eventually, she tricked him into giving her the stone and married another man.

Tiger's eye is considered sacred by some tribes and can only be worn or carried by those deemed worthy. It has also been auspicious symbol for weddings and new beginnings.

Amber

Native Americans have used healing crystals and rocks for centuries to promote physical, emotional, and spiritual well-being. These natural resources are believed to have powerful energies that can help to restore balance and harmony in the user's life.

Amber is a fossilized resin often used as a healing stone due to its astringent properties. Amber can help clarify mental and emotional issues, helping to clear blockages in the energy system, and soothing painful emotions. It can also be a protective charm against negative energy and harmful spells.

Other popular stones used by Native Americans for healing purposes include turquoise, quartzite, tiger's eye, amethyst, peridot, topaz, bone china, tourmaline, opal, jadeite, and pearls. Each has unique powers and benefits that can be harnessed by the user to improve their health and well-being.

Carnelian

Carnelian is a type of chalcedony, and it's considered to be one of the most spiritual healing stones. Indigenous people in North America used carnelian to heal physical and emotional wounds. It was also thought to enhance psychic abilities and provide protection from harm. Carnelian is known for clearing energy blockages and facilitating positive change.

Howlite

Howlite is a variety of chalcedony and fluorite. It is found in many colors, but most often, it is white or light-colored with black speckles. It has been used by Native Americans for centuries as a healing crystal and rock.

Native Americans believe that howlite helps connect people to the spiritual world and strengthens relationships. They use howlite to clear energy blockages, increase concentration and clarity of thought, and promote peace.

Howlite is also known for its ability to heal physical ailments. It can help reduce pain, ease inflammation, and boost the immune system.

Leopard Skin Jasper

Native Americans have long been known for their healing crystals and rocks. Many people turn to these natural resources to help heal themselves and their loved ones. Leopard skin Jasper is a popular choice for those looking for a helpful stone.

Leopard skin Jasper is said to be especially beneficial for calming and soothing the mind and emotions. It is also believed to promote inner peace and help clear blocked energy channels. This stone can also be very helpful when addressing physical issues such as pain relief, inflammation, and stress relief.

Leopard skin Jasper may be a great option if you're looking for an all-around healing crystal that can support your overall health and well-being.

Pyrite

Pyrite is a stone used for centuries by Native American tribes. It is said to have healing properties and can be used to improve vision, fertility, and protection from negative energy. Some of the other stones that are often used in conjunction with pyrite include turquoise, amethyst, topaz, and onyx.

Snowflake Obsidian

Obsidian is popular for healing crystals and rocks among Native American tribes. The obsidian is found in many different colors. Still, the snowflake variety is especially prized because it is said to have properties that help heal the mind, body, and spirit.

Obsidian is thought to have natural abilities to focus spiritual energy and cleanse and energize the Chakras. It has been used by indigenous people for centuries as a tool for healing, meditation, and communication with the spirit world.

The hunters who find obsidian often use it to make tools, ornaments, and ceremonial items such as knives or pipes. Because of its sharp edges and transparency, obsidian is also used in artistry to create beautiful jewelry pieces.

Book 10:
Native American Herbal Gardening

Chapter 1: Gardening And Herbalist Tools To Have
Main Gardening Tools

While building your library, you can take the next baby step of growing your herbs. Or it could be a small window herb garden in your home. The choice depends on your level of comfortableness with the idea.

Perhaps, you are already growing herbs for culinary purposes. I know Grace always had parsley available for healing and to throw into her delicious soups. Whenever I visited her, I left with a handful of parsley or basil. If you are already growing these, you're already a budding herbalist.

What you decide to grow will depend on a few factors. If you're considering an outside garden, you need to find out what will thrive in your climate. Call your local county extension service if you can't get the answers you need from an online search.

Once you know what herbs to grow, you need to increase your chances of success by seeking advice on the soil, sunlight, and other growth requirements.

Gardening can be a lot of work, but it's also very rewarding to see your plants grow and produce fruits and vegetables. To make the process as simple and enjoyable as possible, ensure you have the right tools.

My husband spent a lot of time introducing me to the various tools of the trade. Each gardening tool is more important than the last and has a significant role in the gardening field.

This chapter will introduce you to the different and most important tools you should know about when starting your gardening journey.

Spade

If you garden, you need a spade. A spade is one of the most important tools a gardener has. It's the perfect tool for breaking up the soil and turning over the Earth to uncover new plants and flowers. A good spade will also be able to handle roots and smaller rocks. Here are five must-have spades for any gardener:

Hoe

The hoe is another classic garden tool that has been in use for centuries. Hoes are similar in shape to spades but usually have a more pointed end. They're ideal for soft soils and can loosen soil, remove weeds, and cultivate gardens. It should only be used with soft soils, as they can damage hard surfaces.

Trowel

A trowel is one of the most important tools a gardener can have. It helps you turn the soil, break up compacted materials, and shape plants. A good trowel has a long handle that is comfortable to grip and a sharp blade at the end.

Soil Knife

Simply put, a soil knife is essential for removing dried-out or compacted soil from your garden bed. Not only does this help improve the performance of your plants, but it also helps to maintain healthy soils and prevent root rot.

Lawn Rake

Rakes are great for removing leaves, debris, and snow from your lawn. They are also perfect for grooming flower beds and trimming hedges.

Spading Fork

This simple tool is essential for moving soil and breaking up clumps. It's also useful for removing large rocks or roots from the ground.

Hoe Fork

These allow you to Till and cultivate your garden precisely, making it easier for you to get the most out of your plants. Hoe forks come in various sizes and shapes, so you're sure to find one that suits your needs.

Hand Scythe

A hand scythe is a versatile tool that can be used for various tasks in the garden. It is great for cutting down long grass and weeds and hacking away at smaller plants. A hand scythe can also be used to harvest fruits and vegetables and trim hedges and other vegetation.

There are a few things to consider when choosing a hand scythe. The blade should be sharp, and the handle should be comfortable. The blade should also be adjustable to accommodate different cutting tasks.

Scuffle Hoe

A scuffle hoe is a gardening tool that helps loosen soil and remove weeds. It is also known as a weed shredder, cultivator, or hoe-shovel. This tool has a long metal handle with a V-shaped blade on one end and tines on the other. It scrapes the soil's surface, removing weeds and unwanted plants.

Stake Rod

When gardening, it is important to use a stake rod to secure plants in place. A stake rod helps keep plants from moving, keeps them from toppling over, and makes it easier to lift plants. There are many different types of stake rods available on the market, so choosing one compatible with your gardening tools and the type of garden you are working in is important.

Pruning Saw

A pruning saw helps trim and remove branches, shrubs, and other plants. You can use it to clean up trees and plants in your garden. You can also use it to cut flowers and other plants.

Broom

A broom sweeps debris and bugs off the soil's surface, preventing them from nesting and damaging plants. Effective broom use also aerates and makes sure that there is adequate moisture in the soil.

Watering Can

A watering can is an essential tool for any gardener. Not only does it help you to water your plants more efficiently, but it also makes it easier to avoid wetting your feet. There are a variety of watering cans available on the market, so it's important to choose the right one for your needs.

One of the most important factors to consider when purchasing a watering can is the water reservoir size. Some reservoirs hold up to three gallons of water, while others hold only one gallon. If you plan on using your watering can extensively, it's important to get a reservoir that holds enough water.

Another important factor to consider when purchasing a watering can is the type of hose connector included. Some cans have connectors that fit into standard garden hoses. In contrast, others have connectors that fit into specialized hoses designed for gardening. It's important to choose a watering can with a connector that will work with the type of hose that you have.

Finally, make sure to check out the reviews of the watering cans that are available on the market. Reviews can help you to determine which watering can is best suited for your needs.

Some additional ones that you may need include:

- Pruning sheers
- Garden Scissors
- Hand Hoe
- Mower
- Cultivator
- Wheelbarrow

Essential Tools For Herbalists

As a herbalist, you are likely familiar with "herbalism." But what does it really mean? What are the essential tools of the trade? And how do they help you to provide your patients with the best possible care? In this section, we will explore the basics of herbalism and discuss the essential tools every herbalist should have in their kit. From therapeutic plants to essential equipment, read on to learn more about the tools that will help you provide the best possible care for your patients.

Scissors And Baskets

If you're a herbalist, you know that scissors and baskets are essential tools for your work. Scissors are used to cut herbs and other plants, while baskets can store herbs after they have been cut.

Scissors should always be sharpened, and it is important to use the right size for the task. For example, if you're cutting large chunks of herbs, you'll need a larger pair of scissors than cutting small pieces. Baskets can also be customized in various ways to make them more efficient for your work. For example, some herbalists prefer baskets with wide mouths that allow them to easily pick up large quantities of herbs. In contrast, others prefer smaller baskets that can be carried around more easily.

Mesh Sieve

A Mesh sieve is used in herbalism and aromatherapy to strain plant material, usually flowers or leaves. It typically has a fine mesh surface and can be made from various materials, including cotton, silk, or gauze.

Mesh sieves are often used in conjunction with other tools for herb gatherings, such as a basket or collection jar. They allow for the removal of smaller particles from the plant material, which can help to improve the quality and potency of the final product.

Potato Ricer

It's true, if odd, an odd necessity for an herbal student. But a potato ricer is indispensable. I use this instead of the more expensive tincture press. The press and my ricer apply pressure to the tincture to remove all the liquid from the herbs.

Mortar And Pestle

When it comes to herbalism, every healer should have a few essential tools on hand. One of these is a mortar and pestle. This simple tool can create finely powdered blends and soups and stews.

A mortar and pestle are typically made from hardwood or stone and come with a bowl on one end and a pestle on the other. The user puts the ingredients into the bowl, grinding them together until they form a paste or powder. This is an easy way to create herbs in bulk or to finely grind spices for cooking.

The pestle can also crush seeds or fruits for mixing into smoothies or juices. And since many herbs contain volatile oils that can irritate the nose and throat, using a mortar and pestle will help you to avoid those unpleasant side effects.

So if you're looking for an easy way to get started in herbalism, keep a mortar and pestle handy!

Spice Grinder

A spice grinder can be a very useful tool for a herbalist. It allows you to grind up dried herbs, spices, and other ingredients for your cooking or herbal remedies. There are many different types of spice grinders on the market, so choosing one that will fit your needs is important.

Some typical features of a spice grinder include a secure lid that prevents herbs from spilling during use, an easily removable grinding mechanism, and a hopper capacity that accommodates a variety of ground herbs. Some models also have variable speeds to allow you to control the fineness of the powder.

Before buying a spice grinder, read reviews online and compare different models. You should also consider how often you plan to use the grinder and what type of spices or herbs you will use it for.

Canning Jars

Canning jars are essential tools for any herbalist. They can be used for storing dried herbs, making tinctures and potions, and canning fruits and vegetables.

While various types of canning jars are available, the most popular type is the wide-mouth jar. This jar has a large opening at the top that makes it easy to fill with ingredients and remove them from the jar after they have been canned.

A thick wall design and a secure seal are other important features when selecting canning jars. The wall should be thick enough to resist shattering during high-pressure canning but not so thick that it becomes difficult to clean. A good seal prevents oxygen from entering the jar and the spoilage of the contents.

Kitchen Scale

A kitchen scale can be an essential tool for any herbalist. It is useful for weighing herbs and other ingredients. It can also make precise measurements when mixing herbal remedies or tinctures. There are a variety of scales available on the market, so it's important to find one that fits your needs.

Some scales have multiple weighing modes, such as ounces or grams, while others only have one. It's also important to look for a scale with a large capacity; some models have capacities of up to 10 pounds. Finally, ensure the scale has a good readout; ideally, it should display grams and ounces.

Tea Press

Like my potato ricer, this is one of my favorite herbal instruments. It makes brewing large amounts of tea so much easier. It's also great to use when you make infusions. If all you have at home is a coffee press, then use that. It serves the same purpose. But just a word of caution is in order. It's best to have one that's dedicated to your herbal avocation. That way, your teas won't have any lingering coffee taste.

Tea Strainer

A tea strainer is a perfect appliance for only one cup of tea.

Electric Teapot

Electric teapots are a great way to make tea quickly and easily. They come in various sizes, so you can find one that fits your needs. Some electric teapots have timers so you can preset the time for your tea, and others have alarms that let you know when the tea is ready. Electric teapots are also easy to clean, so you'll never have to worry about making a mess in your kitchen again.

Knife

Knives come in all shapes and sizes and can be purchased for various purposes. For many herbalists, knives are an essential tool for harvesting plants. There are a few key types of knives that herbalists should have on hand:

-A Herbalist's Knife: This type of knife is designed to harvest plants. It has a long blade that is often curved or serrated, making it easier to cut through thick branches.

-A scalpel: A scalpel is similar to a hermit knife but is smaller and designed for use on finer plant material.

-A garden shear: Garden shears are typically used to cut stems or leaves from plants. They come in various shapes and sizes, so select the correct model for your needs.

Cutting Board

A quality cutting board is essential for any herbalist, and various options are available on the market. Some boards are made of wood, while others are made from food-grade plastic.

Whichever type of cutting board you choose, make sure to keep the following in mind:

1. size - the cutting board should be large enough to accommodate your knives and ingredients comfortably but not so large as to become a cluttered workspace.

2. material - choose a cutting board that is both durable and easy to clean. Wood boards can stain easily, while plastic boards are often easier to keep clean.

3. design - find a cutting board that fits your aesthetic preferences, whether sleek or rustic. There are also many unique and stylish cutting boards available today.

Double Boiler

If you're a herbalist, chances are you've heard of double boiling. Double boiling is used in many traditional healing methods to kill bacteria and other microbes. It's also a great way to make potions and tinctures more potent. Here's how it works:

1. Fill a large pot with water and set it to boil
2. Put the herbs or other ingredients you want to treat into a small, heat-resistant container (like a glass jar or an earthenware mug) and put this container into the boiling water
3. Reduce the heat to low and let the mixture simmer for about 20 minutes
4. Carefully remove the small container from the pot of boiling water and set it aside on cool ground or in an ice bath
5. Pour out all of the liquid from the small container into another pot or bowl
6. Return the small container filled with herbs or other ingredients to the pot of hot water, making sure that it is submerged
7. Boil this liquid for 5 minutes, then carefully pour it out onto the cool ground or into an ice bath

Measuring Spoon And Cups

If you are a herbalist, then measuring spoons and cups are essential tools for your work. These can be used to measure dry herbs or liquids and come in different sizes to accommodate any need.

When selecting a measuring spoon, think about the factors that will be most important to you. Some of these factors include the material the spoon is made from (e.g., stainless steel), the shape of the spoon, and how easy it is to hold and use.

Cups can also be important for herbalists. Different types of cups are available, including ceramic cups that can withstand high temperatures and silicone cups that are non-toxic and flexible enough to fit many different shapes. It's important to select a cup appropriate for the herbs you will be working with; for example, if you are measuring dried herbs, choose a cup made from porcelain rather than plastic.

When measuring liquids, it's important to take into account the volume of the liquid as well as its temperature. For example, if you are measuring honey at room temperature, use a smaller cup than if it is hot off the stovetop. Similarly, if you're using hot water to make tea, use a larger mug instead of a small cup because hot water takes up more space in a smaller mug than in a larger one.

Finally, wash your measuring spoons and cups before using them to avoid contamination.

Large Mixing Bowls

Looking for the perfect large mixing bowl? Look no further! These bowls are perfect for herbalists and have a variety of uses. They can mix ingredients, store dried herbs, or even serve food.

One popular option is the stainless steel bowl from KitchenAid. This durable and attractive bowl makes it a great choice for any kitchen. It also has an ergonomic design that makes it easy to work with.

Another great option is the glass bowl from Amazon. This bowl is resistant to heat and cold, making it ideal for storing delicate herbs or spices. It also has a comfortable silicone grip on the bottom, making it easy to move around your kitchen.

If you need a larger mixing bowl that can handle more ingredients, consider the ceramic bowl from Nordic Ware. This bowl is both beautiful and functional, making it a great choice for anyone looking for an upscale option. It also features a non-stick surface, so you can easily mix your ingredients without losing moisture or flavor.

Chapter 2: The Two Types Of Beginner-Friendly Gardens

As you can already tell by now, there are a wide variety of garden types. However, if you are a beginner, I recommend starting with either Raised Bed Gardening or Container Gardening. The remainder of the book will go deep into these two types of gardens and explain how you can set them up to your heart's content. Below I have given a brief breakdown of why I chose these two gardens for this book.

Why Container Gardening Is Beginner Friendly

Few things are more satisfying than watching those tiny seeds you planted not long ago slowly emerge from the Earth to form nourishing vitamin-rich food for you and those you care about. Unfortunately, not everyone in this day and age has a large backyard with soil suitable for growing vegetables. Some of us don't even have a yard! Even the smallest patio, back porch, balcony, or doorstep can accommodate a beautiful and productive container garden.

Planting in pots has a long history that dates back to the first Egyptian, Roman, and Oriental civilizations. The Hanging Gardens of Babylon were considered one of the Seven Wonders of the World, and Henry VIII was so taken with the Hampton Court Gardens that he had its owner arrested and claimed it for himself.

Container Gardening Is Very Simple And Easy

Container gardening is perfect for beginners because it's simple and easy. All you need is a container, some plants, and some soil. You can even buy pre-made containers at most garden stores or use empty food or beverage containers that you can purchase at the grocery store. Once you have your container, fill it with soil and plant your plants. You will then water them and care for them like any other plants in your garden. Container gardening is a great way to get started in gardening, and it's also a great way to keep your garden organized and easy to care for.

Provides A Wide Variety Of Options

Container gardening is perfect for beginners because it's simple to set up and manage. You can start with a small container and grow into a larger garden as you learn the ropes. There are a wide variety of container gardens that you can choose from, so you can find one that fits your style.

Some popular container gardens include vertical gardens, 12-pack gardens, herb gardens, and succulent gardens. Vertical gardens are great for people with limited space because they take up very little space. They are also easy to maintain because all you need to do is water the plants. 12-pack gardens are perfect for people with a lot of space. Still, they don't want to spend hours planting and watering plants individually. Herb gardens are great for people who want to add fresh herbs to their cooking or some fragrance to their home. Succulent gardens are perfect for people who want to add some greenery to their homes but don't have a lot of room. They take up very little space and can be easily watered.

Container Gardening Requires Less Water Than Traditional Gardening

Container gardening is the perfect way to learn how to garden without wasting water. You can plant in smaller doses with a container, preventing excess water from evaporating and wasting. Additionally, you need only a fraction of the space for traditional gardening methods. Finally, containers make it easy to move your plants around as you change your mind about where they should be placed.

Container Gardening Requires Less Water

Container gardening is the perfect way to learn how to garden without wasting water. You can plant in smaller doses with a container, preventing excess water from evaporating and wasting. Additionally, you need only a fraction of the space for traditional gardening methods. Finally, containers make it easy to move your plants around as you change your mind about where they should be placed.

You Can Garden Wherever You Want

Seasoned outdoor gardeners frequently report having an insatiable desire to get started at the start of the planting season. Depending on where you live, the time may differ. It is usually at the approach of winter and the first stirrings of life beneath the frozen ground in temperate regions. However, in the tropics, the fresh smell of Earth pervades the air following the first shower hitting the sun-baked Earth at the start of the rainy season. On the other hand, those who enjoy container gardening do not need to wait for such external cues.

With containers, you can start your garden anytime and on any day – especially if you can cover the container to create a mini greenhouse. There is no need to wait for extremely warm weather to start young plants when a container can be used to create ideal growing conditions.

No Space-Related Issues

You may believe you do not have enough space for a vegetable garden. While people who live in townhouses and apartments may lack outdoor space, this should not be a problem if you turn to container gardening.

Container gardens are not limited by yard space availability (or lack thereof). There is no need for a yard. Many plants can grow on a balcony, a window sill, or a bright spot near a window. Remember that many different plant varieties can be grown in the same container. Companion planting in containers is a popular idea that produces a high yield and allows most people to garden.

Perfect For Inexperienced Gardeners

There are some harsh realities associated with in-ground outdoor gardening. The first is about weeds. Their seeds are everywhere and sprout and grow faster than we plant. That is why experienced gardeners place a high value, time, and effort into preparing the veggie bed. People who take it easy and plant their gardens with little preparation risk having their beds overrun with weeds in no time. This is extremely discouraging, especially for inexperienced gardeners.

Other factors that can harm outdoor gardens include pests, diseases, and natural occurrences. Many inexperienced gardeners are discouraged by their failure and never try gardening again. Although there are risks associated with container gardening, they are minor. Weeds are infrequent, and diseases and pests are easily detected and remedied. Because containers are portable, they can be moved to safer locations when there is a threat of prolonged bad weather.

No-Till Gardening

Even the most ardent outdoor gardener will admit that tilling the soil is back-breaking. Furthermore, it has been discovered that tilling disturbs many of the natural organisms required for a healthy garden. For this reason, many people are opting for a no-till garden.

Container gardening allows you to create a suitable growing environment full of healthy components without having to amend the soil or worry about tilling damage.

Saves Money On Fertilizer

When it comes to feeding, container-grown plants require less frequent fertilizer applications. Fertilizers applied to potted plants, whether chemical or organic, last longer because they remain concentrated in the limited amount of soil within the containers, just like water. Furthermore, potted plants do not need to share fertilizer with competing weeds. Fertilizers should be used sparingly in pots as opposed to garden beds for the same reasons, as high concentrations can burn the roots. Use a high-quality organic fertilizer or make your own compost. You will save money on fertilizer and get more bang for your buck.

Simple Pest Control

Because you don't have access to individual plants, pest infestations in garden beds frequently necessitate pesticide spraying. Pest control in container-grown plants is simpler and may not require chemicals.

Aphids and scale insects can be removed by handpicking the larger insects and using a toothbrush or cotton bud dipped in rubbing alcohol. Moving the pots to the bathroom for an occasional shower is another great way to eliminate many insect pests in the plant's tender parts. Individual pots can even be dipped in tepid water to drown unwanted soil organisms. Keeping the pot in a water plate can keep ants from entering and establishing aphid farms on your prized plants. Slugs and other soft-bodied pests would be deterred by a layer of diatomaceous Earth around the pot.

Harvesting Is Very Simple

Growing vegetables and fruits in containers make harvesting much easier. In pots, grow strawberries, blueberries, and root tubers such as carrots, radishes, potatoes, and sweet potatoes. Instead of digging them up and potentially damaging the valuable produce, simply overturn the pots on a plastic sheet when they are ready for harvest. Shake the soil to ensure that every tuber is in perfect condition.

You Can Adjust The Growing Conditions

Providing the best environment for your container plants is simple without extensive soil amendments. You can give your rhododendrons and blueberries a slightly acidic medium without disturbing the pH of the soil in other containers or garden beds.

Plants can be rearranged according to seasonal differences in light intensity. Plants with similar watering requirements can coexist as long as they are housed in different containers.

You Can Do Quick Makeovers

By simply changing the containers in your garden, you can change the look and theme of your garden. Large stone containers in various architectural shapes, for example, can give the garden a classic look and feel. In contrast, metal containers with copper patina or rust––whether real or fake––can transport you to another time and age. Acrylic containers in jewel colors can add color to your garden. Still, a monochromatic scheme with the same material can be elegant.

Suppose you're interested in starting a garden but don't know where to start. In that case, container gardening may be the perfect solution for you. It is easy to get started, but you can customize your garden to fit your specific needs and preferences. Plus, if you have limited space or are concerned about the weather conditions in your area, container gardening can be a great option.

Why Raised Bed Gardening Is Beginner Friendly

Raised bed gardening is perfect for beginners because it's easy to set up, relatively low-maintenance, and yields a great harvest. A raised bed is a large container filled with soil and then raised on legs or poles. This makes it easy to reach into the bed to dig up plants and keeps weeds from growing between them. You can buy a pre-made raised bed or build your own using materials like lumber, PVC pipe, or stone.

No-Till Gardening

A raised bed prepares your soil for the simplest possible gardening—the 'no work' kind. Gardeners usually maintain their raised beds by adding materials on top rather than tilling up the soil yearly to add fertilizer and amendments. Bush beans grow in a bed with seaweed mulch on top for nutrients and weed suppression.

Compost, mulches, manures, and other soil conditioners can be applied directly to the top few inches of soil without needing arduous labor. And, as worms and roots push their way through, the soil can do its tilling. While regular human tilling depletes the soil structure, doing nothing increases the organic component of your soil over time.

Won't Break Your Back

It's surprising how much back and knee strain can occur simply by weeding a garden, especially a large one, which can have serious long-term consequences. A raised bed, particularly one at least 12 inches tall, can alleviate debilitating back and joint pain. Even young people interested in farming as a career should consider the potential back damage that organic farming can cause through hand weeding. Consider raised beds to be a health-related investment.

More Appealing

Although it may appear pure vanity, having nicer beds can serve a practical purpose. In the city, a raised bed may be necessary to keep your neighbors happy, especially if you want to grow vegetables in your front yard. Raised beds also make pathways easier to maintain because there is a clear line between the bed and the path.

Raised Beds Keeps Pest And Critters Away

Slugs can climb, but the tall sides of a raised garden box slow them down and provide a place to stop them. According to many gardeners, Slugs will not crawl over the copper flashing, which can be used to border your box. You can also cover the bottom of the box with hardware cloth to keep crawling critters like groundhogs from stealing root crops. Dogs are also less likely to urinate directly on your plants due to their height. If deer are a problem, you can add deer fencing directly to your bed or buy a box with a built-in deer fence. It's also much easier to incorporate plastic hoops into raised garden beds for bird barriers, cold frames, or row covers.

Raising Helps With Drainage

A raised garden bed may be the only way to have a full growing season in areas prone to flooding or marshy yards. The most common raised bed depth is 11″, which is one inch below the sides of a 12″ high garden box. This is adequate drainage for most crops and provides plants with nearly a foot of extra breathing space above wet conditions. Raised beds also drain better in general, even when it rains heavily.

Lots Of Ergonomic Options

These containers allow you to build higher-level beds, reducing the back, neck, and shoulder strain commonly associated with traditional non-container gardening practices.

Physical strain is the most discouraging factor for both new and experienced gardeners. On the other hand, raised beds can help you get over that hump and keep your enthusiasm for gardening alive – rather than feeling tired and hurt every time you think about it!

Easy Weed Control

By keeping your garden's earthy contents separate from the wild surroundings outside its comfortable container, you reduce the possibility of weed seeds spreading through your growing environment and, thus, weed growth.

Because you're bringing in your own mix, to begin with, you're doubling your protection against weed invasion, especially if your soil mix is weed-free.

Last but not least, if your kit or construction includes bottom protection that protects against the Earth beneath it, it will be even more difficult for plants and weeds growing outside the container to get in!

Increased Root Growth

Low-set containers with ground contact – and/or that hold a finer-textured growing mix – allow for faster root development than plants planted in backyard sod or hard-pan alone.

Such soils are more difficult for root development and impact plant appearance, health, and harvest times. Not if you use your own mix, especially one better suited to nurturing sensitive plant growth.

According to the University of Missouri Extension, better root growth equals healthier plants and higher yields!

Less Compaction of the Soil

Because the soil in containers is never compacted by being walked on, it is ideal for both plant and soil health. Sheltered kits can help reduce compaction by providing shelter from heavy rain.

Many of my farmer mentors have told me, "compacted soil is the bane of all growers!" An elevated container almost guarantees that this cunning obstacle will never be your enemy again.

According to the University of Georgia Cooperative Extension, it's a wise addition to your garden, especially if there is high foot traffic (and the presence of less careful, rambunctious children) nearby.

Increased Yields

The appeal of increasing vegetable and produce yields through intensive plantings is a real plus for gardeners who want to grow their own food.

Raised beds are ideal for much closer-clustered plantings, such as in square-foot gardening, bio-intensive planting, and other styles.

Instead of having a traditional garden with many paths or spaces for conventional row planting, you use up ALL of your space in a much smaller container garden. You can thus grow a lot more in only a fraction of the space.

Chapter 3: The Process Of Preparation And Planting Your Herbs
Proper Location

First and foremost, when it comes to locating a suitable place. This is because most herbs require plenty of sunshine to grow healthy and reach their full potential. So before you start preparing your land, you should first observe it and note the sunny spots and how long they shine on your garden. Knowing this will help you grow your herbs in a more efficient place. If you encounter warm summers, you can plant in an area that receives morning sun and afternoon shade. However, other herbs are shade lovers. However, very few of them are good for cooking apart from parsley.

Your herb garden is also intended to be admired, so you should grow it outside your backdoor or in front of your yard. Herbs are tremendously attractive and will make a lovely display, not forgetting the savory scents you will get every time you walk past them. A nearby garden will also enable you to easily access your culinary herbs whenever you need them.

Preparing the Soil

Herbs are easy plants to grow, but that does not mean you can just grow them anywhere. When growing herbs, you must ensure that they have access to well-drained soil that is light and simple to work with. This is because herbs grow better in well-drained soil. How will you know your soil is well-drained? Simply run water in your garden for several minutes using a hose pipe or other tool. If the water puddles up, your soil is not well-drained and needs amends. You can improve it by adding compost, peat, and soil. Be careful when adding compost; if you mistake overdoing it, it will make your soil too rich, which can result in your herbs being prone to diseases and cause them to be weak.

The best soil for growing herbs is loamy soil that consists of sand, silt, organic matter, and clay. This type of soil contains quantities of potash, phosphorous, nitrogen, and trace elements necessary for promoting good growth. But what if you don't have this type of soil in your garden? You can still use the type of soil you have after improving its quality to fit that one of loamy soil. Adding organic materials to clay soil (for example, compost, coarse sand, green hummus, peat moss, and well-aged chicken or cow dung) may help to improve its structure and fertility. The combination of these organic materials gives your soil friability.

Testing your soil helps you to analyze the soil PH, which is a very important factor. Having acidic or alkaline soil might prevent nutrients from reaching your plant if they are not properly circulated in the soil. Most herbs require a neutral soil PH, which ranges from 6.5 to 7.5. So how can you determine your soil PH? Take a few samples, preferably 2 cups of soil from different areas of your garden, then take it to your testing facility, which can be your local county extension, gardening companies, and independent labs. Once the results are in, add Sulphur if your PH results are higher than 7.3 and add agricultural lime if your soil PH is lower than 6.5 to balance your soil PH.

Planting Herbs

When it comes to planting herbs, you need around 8 inches in diameter for each plant. Guidelines you will need for growing different herbs:

- 1 foot- Parsley, Dill, Chives, Cilantro
- 2 feet- Savory, Tarragon, Thyme, Basils
- 3-4 feet- Marjoram, Oregano, Mints, Sage, Rosemary.

Once you have the required feet of the type of herbs you want to plant, start planting by following the below steps:

1. Start digging your garden with a large fork to loosen the soil, which has become condensed for some years. This improves the drainage system by allowing the water to penetrate the soil and creating space for plant roots to spread into the soil.
2. The next step is to add some compost, i.e., an inch on top of your garden soil, and then mix it up. This will help your soil by increasing its nutrient content in it as well as improving its drainage.
3. Take a trowel and prepare some trenches for seeding. Bear in mind you can also use your hands if you don't have a trowel.
4. Next, take your seeds and swiftly scatter them down the trenches as you try and achieve the recommended spacing. You can also mix sand with the seeds to make them easier to handle.
5. Finally, cover the seeds lightly with the soil and then water them until they are wet. You shouldn't be worried if you are overseeding during scattering. You can thin your plants later if they are too many for your liking.

Mulching

Mulching is simply covering the surface of your cultivated soil with sheets of materials. Mulching makes your garden neat, but that's not all; it also improves the soil around your plants and minimizes the time spent on weeding and watering. That's why your next step is to put a 3-4 inch layer of mulch onto your garden so that it can reduce the need for cultivation and weeding.

Watering

Herbs require a relatively high amount of water. So if there is no rain, you will need to occasionally supply your herb garden with water. You must soak your garden once or twice a week when watering herbs. The best equipment to use when it comes to watering herbs is a soaker hose. This is because it is easier for you to soak the plants with 1 inch of water, which herbs need once per week to grow efficiently when using a soaker hose. The amount of water needed changes when in hot and dry conditions and when your plants are actively growing. The two conditions will require you to increase your water supply since evaporation rate is high.

Word of caution: you should avoid sprinkling water lightly into your garden, as it will force the roots of the herbs to the surface.

The other method which you can use to water herbs is drip irrigation. This method significantly reduces the amount of water lost through evaporation which is perfect for growing herbs. The type of soil used in your garden also matters when it comes to watering. If you use sandy soil, you will need to water your herbs more than when you use heavier soil.

Staking

When growing your herbs, you may find some of them weak enough to stand on their own. These plants need you to stake them, i.e., support them to shoot up comfortably. You will need to have different sizes of stakes in your garden. You can use bamboo sticks; use a good number of them to tie a tall plant with them using raffia or green tape. The herb will grow through the grid and eventually cover the supporting sticks completely. For the best stake, you will need to find one that doesn't interfere with the growth of the herbs. A good example of less conspicuous staking is a metal ring with a grind inside.

Word of advice: You should start placing a staking system before your herbs become too tall. The plants will grow more naturally when you stake them early.

Weeding

As long as you water your herbs and give them enough nutrients, weeds will always grow, as those are their ideal conditions for growing. Therefore, they will come and fight for nutrients and moisture that your herbs are getting from the soil. Still, unfortunately, this will only limit the healthy growth of your herbs. That's why you should make sure you occasionally inspect your garden and prune out all the weeds for your herbs to grow without straining resources. Weeds can be perennial, annual, or biennial. If you have a small garden (which I believe you are just starting), the best approach is to uproot the weeds by hand after watering the soil.

Harvesting and Storing

Once the plants are ready for harvesting, pick the leaves or flowers with your fingers, or snip them with kitchen shears for a cleaner harvest. Pick the mature stalks and flowers at the top of the plant, and do not pick the stems bare. You want to allow the plants to regrow. It is best to harvest the herbs when you want to use them to ensure freshness. Wash them thoroughly to remove bugs, dirt, and soil. If you need to store herbs later, you can dry or freeze them. You must wash them gently and remove excess water by patting them with a paper towel.

To dry herbs, cut the stems at soil level, tie a bunch together at the bottom of the stem, and hang them upside down to dry for y week or two. Once dried, remove the leaves or flowers from the stem and store them in a dry, airtight container. This way, they should last for a year. Dried herbs make excellent teas and food seasoning.

To freeze herbs, chop up the clean herbs and place teaspoons full into an ice cube tray cells. Fill the tray with water and freeze. The benefit of freezing is that herbs retain their just-picked flavor. Pop out an ice cube and put it into a pot or cup like you would do with fresh herbs when needed.

Chapter 4: Tips On How To Grow Herbs In Your Garden

Gardening can be a rewarding experience, whether you're growing fresh produce or flowers. But if you want to spruce up your garden without spending a fortune, there are a few things you need to know. This section will provide tips on how to grow herbs in your garden, from selecting the right plants to watering and fertilizing them. We will also give you tips on creating the perfect environment for growing herbs so they can flourish and bring flavor to your meals.

A General Overview

Growing your own is definitely the way to go if you're looking to add a little spice to your cooking or enjoy fresh herbs. Not only are herbs easy to grow, but they also provide numerous health benefits. Here are six tips for growing herbs in your garden:

1. Choose the right location: Herbs prefer well-drained soil with plenty of sun and water.

2. Plant them early: Herb seeds should be planted outdoors as soon as the ground can be worked in early Spring, before the first frost.
3. Mulch them: Apply a layer of mulch over the herb plants after planting to help keep moisture and weeds at bay.
4. Harvest regularly: Harvest herbs when actively producing flowers (usually around 6 weeks after planting), then trim off dead leaves and flowers.
5. Propagate from cuttings: Take cuttings from mature plants and propagate them in moist sponges or perlite before inserting them into the soil again.

Plant Your Herbs In Well Draining Soil

There are several ways to grow herbs in your garden, but growing them in well-draining soil is the most popular. Planting herbs in a raised bed or in containers reduces water requirements and helps keep the soil moist.

To amend your soil for herb gardening, test it for pH levels and add lime if needed. Add organic matter such as compost or aged manure when preparing the soil. Add water slowly until the surface of the soil is moist but not wet. Check the water level daily for container plants and top off as needed.

Here are some tips for planting herbs:

1. Choose a sunny spot with good drainage where your herbs can get plenty of light.
2. Choose a mix of hardy and tender varieties of plants suited to your climate and garden space. Many plants can be grown in containers outdoors during warm months, brought inside during the cooler months, or planted directly into the ground in colder climates.
3. Space plants evenly so they have room to grow tall; a dense arrangement can lead to nutrient deficiencies and fungal overgrowth. When transplanting young plants, gently break up large clumps with your hands before replanting them into individual pots or cells.

Lightly Fertilise Your Herbs

One of the quickest and easiest ways to grow your own herbs is to lightly fertilize them once a month. This will help increase their growth rate and ensure they remain healthy and vibrant. Here are some tips on how to fertilize your herbs:

1. Add a light layer of compost or manure to the soil around your herb plants. This will provide them with the nutrients they need to grow vigorously.

2. When using natural methods such as composting, add some nitrogen-rich organic matter, such as green leaves or straw, when you mix it in. Nitrogen is essential for plant growth, so adding these extras will help make sure that your herbs get all the nutrients they need.

3. If using artificial fertilizers, make sure they are diluted before applying them to the soil around your herb plants. Over-fertilising can cause damage to both the plants and the environment, so you must take care when doing this.

Plant And Group Similar Herbs Together

Like most gardeners, you're probably familiar with growing a few common herbs, such as parsley, rosemary, or Thyme. But what about the hundreds of other herbs available to gardeners? In this section, we'll teach you how to grow 16 common herbs together in your garden!

Basil is a great herb to grow with carrots because they both have a strong flavor and can be used fresh or dried. Thyme and parsley are good companions because they share similar flavors and can be used fresh or dried. Lavender, oregano, and mint are good herb combinations because they all have a strong aroma. Chamomile, hyssop, and lemon balm are good choices for plants that need an easy-to-grow container. Finally, rosemary is a great companion for tomatoes because it helps keep pests away from the plants.

Know The Variety Of Your Herbs And Their Specific Requirements

Herbs are a great way to add flavor and nutrients to your garden, and there are many varieties to choose from. Here are some tips for growing herbs in your garden:

Choose the right variety of herbs. Different herbs have different needs, so choosing the right one for your garden is important. Some most common herb varieties include basil, cilantro, chives, dill, fennel, lavender, mint, oregano, parsley, rosemary, sage, and Thyme.

Cool-weather herbs need more light than warm-weather herbs. Most herbs, like full sun or part sun, will do well in partial shade. Ensure to water them regularly during dry periods and provide fertilizer if needed.

Herbs like garlic mustard require moist soil and lots of organic matter to grow successfully. Add compost or manure before planting these plants. Garlic mustard can also be grown in pots or containers outdoors in warm climates.

Keep Quick-Growing Herbs Apart

Quick-growing herbs like curly parsley, rosemary, and Thyme can easily grow together in the same pot or container if grown in a similar soil type. However, to prevent these herbs from overwhelming each other, it is best to keep quick-growing herbs separate from slower-growing herbs. This can be done by placing them in different pots or containers or growing them in different garden areas.

Plant Your Herbs In Cool Seasons And At The Right Time Depending On The Need

There are a few things to remember when growing herbs in your garden: the climate, the time of year, and the type of herb.

Climate: Herbs prefer cool seasons (between 59-86 degrees Fahrenheit), although they will do well in warm climates too.

Time of Year: Herbs grow best between early Spring and late Fall.

Type of Herb: Herbs can be grown in any soil but are especially fond of dry, sandy soil. They also like full sun or partial shade.

Book 11:
Herbal Recipes
For Your Child's Health

Chapter 1: Common Medicinal Herbs And Their Properties

Medicinal herbs have been used throughout history for both culinary and medicinal purposes. Today, they are still being used to treat a wide variety of ailments, both minor and major. This section will provide you with a guide to some of the most common medicinal herbs, their properties, and how to use them. From headaches to colds and everything in between, this guide will help you get the most out of these natural remedies.

Herbs For Anxiety

Many different herbs have been used for centuries to help with anxiety. Most popular include lavender, chamomile, skullcap, and ginger. Here is a list of some of the most commonly used herbs for anxiety:

Lavender: Lavender is known for its relaxing properties and has been used for centuries to help ease anxiety. It can be taken as a tea or oil infused into skin care products.

Chamomile: Chamomile is also known for its calming effects and has been used in herbal remedies for centuries. It can be brewed as tea or taken as capsules or tablets.

Skullcap: Skullcap is known to help improve cognitive function and reduce anxiety. It can be brewed as tea or taken as capsules or tablets.

Ginger: Ginger effectively treats both physical and mental symptoms of anxiety. It can be eaten fresh or cooked into dishes like gingerbread cookies or soup.

Herbs For Arthritis

Many herbs have been used for centuries to treat arthritis and other conditions. Here are a few of the most popular:

Ginger: Ginger is a natural anti-inflammatory agent and helps relieve pain, stiffness, and inflammation. It can also help to improve joint function. To use ginger medicinally, eat fresh ginger root or ale tea made with ginger root, cloves, and honey.

Cayenne pepper: Cayenne pepper is another natural anti-inflammatory agent that can help reduce joint pain and swelling. To use cayenne pepper medicinally, add it to food or drink as desired. Capsaicin–the main active ingredient in cayenne peppers–can cause minor skin irritation in some people but is generally safe when taken in recommended doses.

Turmeric: Turmeric is a powerful herb used for centuries to treat inflammation and pain throughout the body. Studies suggest that it may also help treat arthritis. To use turmeric medicinally, take capsules or tablets containing ground turmeric mixed with oil (such as olive oil) or water. Also, add ground turmeric to foods such as curries or soups for extra flavor and health benefits.

Herbs For Cancer

Many herbs have been traditionally used to treat cancer. Many of these herbs have been shown in research to have anti-cancer properties. Here is a list of some of the most common herbs used for cancer:

Basil: Basil is effective in treating lung, prostate, and skin cancers. It can also help stop the growth of tumors.

Echinacea: Echinacea is a popular herb for treating cancer because it has anti-tumor properties and can help speed up healing.

Ginger: Ginger has anti-inflammatory properties, which can help reduce cancer symptoms. It is also believed to support the immune system and help eradicate cancer cells.

Goldenseal: Goldenseal is an herbal remedy traditionally used to improve immunity and fight off infection. It has also been shown to be effective in fighting cancerous cells.

Herbs For Colds And Flu

Many herbs can be used for treating colds and flu. These herbs can be taken internally, applied topically to the skin, or mixed with water and drunk as tea. The following is a list of some common medicinal herbs which can be used for treating colds and flu:

Garlic: Garlic has been shown to have antiviral properties, which makes it an effective treatment for colds and flu. Garlic can be taken orally, applied topically to the skin, or mixed with water and drunk as tea.

Ginger: Ginger has also been shown to have antiviral properties, making it an effective treatment for colds and flu. Ginger can be taken orally, applied topically to the skin, or mixed with water and drunk as tea.

Cayenne pepper is also known to have antiviral properties, making it an effective treatment for colds and flu. Cayenne pepper can be taken orally, applied topically to the skin, or mixed with water and drunk as tea.

Herbs For Digestion

If you're looking to improve your digestion, many herbs can help. Here are five herbal supplements that can support regularity and digestion: chamomile (Matricaria chamomilla), ginger (Zingiber officinale), fennel (Foeniculum vulgare), dandelion (Taraxacum officinale), and licorice (Glycyrrhiza glabra).

Chamomile is a versatile herb that is used for a variety of purposes, including digestive support. This flowering plant contains camomile oil, which is reported to help improve intestinal health by enhancing the absorption of nutrients, easing constipation, and reducing inflammation. One cup of chamomile tea daily is enough to relieve digestive issues such as diarrhea and stomach cramps.

Ginger is another popular herb for digestive support. This root-like vegetable has been shown to improve gut health by promoting the growth of beneficial bacteria, resolving inflammation, and reducing pain. In addition to being helpful for digestion, ginger also helps relieve nausea and vomiting due to gastrointestinal illness. To maximize the benefits of ginger for gut health, include it in food or supplement form several times a day.

Fennel is another herb beneficial for digestion. This aromatic vegetable contains an essential oil called anethole, which effectively relieves symptoms of IBS (irritable bowel syndrome.

Herbs For Hormone Imbalance

Many herbs can help to restore balance in the body's hormone system. Some of the most popular herbs for hormone imbalance include:

St. John's wort is a popular herb for restoring balance in the body's hormone system. It has improved symptoms such as depression, anxiety, PMS, and menopausal problems.

Licorice is another herb often used to restore balance in the body's hormone system. Licorice has improved symptoms such as hot flashes, mood swings, osteoporosis, and infertility.

Ashwagandha is a herbal remedy that has been shown to support healthy hormones in both men and women. Ashwagandha has been used traditionally to improve sexual function, stress relief, anxiety relief, and overall well-being.

If you're like most people, you probably don't know much about medicinal herbs. In this guide, we'll help to shed some light on these plants and what they can do for your health. We'll touch on the history of each herb and explain how it can be used to treat various conditions. Finally, we'll provide tips on identifying and purchasing medicinal herbs from trusted sources. By the end of this guide, you will have a basic understanding of the benefits of using medicinal herbs and where to find them.

Chapter 2: The Best Medical Herbs For Kids

Kids have definitely been going through a lot of changes in recent years. There's a lot for them to take in from school to extracurricular activities. That's why it's so important that they get the best possible care possible. And what better way to do that than by using natural remedies? This section will explore some of the best medicinal herbs for kids and how they can help them improve their health. We'll cover things like fever reduction, respiratory relief, and more. So whether you're looking for herbal remedies for yourself or your children, read on for all the details!

Lemon Balm

Lemon balm (Melissa officinalis) is a perennial herb that grows up to one meter tall. The leaves are divided into oblong or elliptical leaflets, and the flowers are small, white, and fragrant. Lemon balm is a well-known remedy for anxiety and stress, as it has been used in folk medicine for centuries.

One of the most important properties of lemon balm is its ability to stimulate the secretion of oxytocin, which is known to reduce stress levels and promote relaxation. Additionally, lemon balm contains menthol and other essential oils that have anti-inflammatory properties. In fact, studies have shown that lemon balm can help reduce pain relief requirements in patients undergoing radiation treatment.

Chamomile

Chamomile is a highly regarded medical herb for treating anxiety, insomnia, and digestive problems. It's also been used to promote relaxation and improve sleep. Chamomile can be brewed as a tea or used in supplements.

Rose

Rose is a folk medicine used for centuries to treat various health problems. Rose oil is known to have healing properties, including treating skin conditions and aiding in wound healing.

Some other benefits of rose oil include reducing anxiety and improving moods. It can also reduce inflammation, help with weight loss, and improve overall circulation. Rose oil is also claimed to help treat psoriasis and eczema.

Spearmint

Spearmint is a perennial herb that is native to Europe and Asia. It grows up to 2 feet tall and has small, narrow leaves that are light green and pointed at the tips. The flowers are small and white and grow in clusters on long stalks.

Spearmint is known for its strong scent, which is said to have health benefits. The oil found in spearmint can help to reduce anxiety and stress, improve cognitive function, and fight inflammation. Additionally, spearmint can promote better breathing thanks to its ability to clear respiratory infections and congestion.

Some potential side effects of taking spearmint supplements include diarrhea, gas, nausea, and vomiting. Therefore, speaking with your healthcare provider before using this herb if you are pregnant or breastfeeding is important.

Marshmallow

Marshmallow is a traditional Chinese herbal medicine that has been used to treat a variety of disorders since ancient times. In recent years, marshmallow has become increasingly popular as a natural remedy for children's health problems. Here are five benefits of using marshmallows for children:

1. Marshmallows can help calm restless children.
2. Marshmallow can help improve attention spans and focus in children with ADHD.
3. Marshmallows can help relieve the symptoms of anxiety and depression in kids.
4. Marshmallow treats kids' respiratory issues, such as bronchitis and pneumonia.
5. Lastly, marshmallow is also useful for treating other childhood ailments, such as diarrhea and indigestion.

Lavender

Lavender is a popular aromatherapy relieves anxiety, stress, headaches, and pain. It can also help treat insomnia, allergies, and cramps. Lavender oil also relieves skin conditions such as eczema and psoriasis.

Violets

Violet is a popular herb for improving mood and relieving anxiety. It has also been used to treat insomnia and depression and regulate blood pressure and heart rate. In addition, violet is believed to help improve cognitive function in children.

Anise

Anise is a spice that comes from an evergreen shrub. The dried fruits of the anise plant are used to make licorice and anise oil, which are used in food and medicine. Anise is also a flavoring in foods, drinks, and pharmaceuticals.

Some medical benefits of anise include reducing inflammation, promoting digestion, and treating gas and flatulence. It can also help relieve anxiety and nervousness, reduce menstrual cramps, lower cholesterol levels, and ease coughs and cold symptoms.

Cinnamon

Cinnamon is a powerful antioxidant shown to help improve blood sugar levels in people with diabetes. It can also help to reduce inflammation and protect the heart. Cinnamon is also thought to have anti-inflammatory and antibacterial properties, which could help treat various conditions, including asthma, Crohn's disease, and ulcerative colitis.

Elder

Elder is a popular herb for treating respiratory problems like bronchitis and pneumonia. It is also beneficial for treating inflammation, infections, and fevers. The fruit of the elder tree is called elderberry. The berries can be eaten fresh or used to make wine, syrup, or jam.

The leaves and flowers of the elder tree are also used medicinally. The leaves can be brewed as a tea to treat cold and flu symptoms, while the flowers can be used as a tea substitute for people who are allergic to other flowers. Elderflower tea has been shown to improve cognitive function in older adults.

Chapter 3: Homemade Herbs Recipes For Kid's Health

Herbal Ginger Brew

This is a great brew for stomach cramps, indigestion, and nausea. It is an energy stimulant used to cure sore throats and coughs.

Ingredients:

- Syrup
- 1/2 cup peeled sliced ginger
- 1 cup water
- 1/4 cup pure maple syrup
- 1 cup carbonated water
- One tablespoon of lemon juice
- Grated lemon, rind

Directions:

1. For the syrup, combine water and ginger in a saucepan, and simmer for 30
1. minutes.
2. Cool slightly and strain.
3. Add maple syrup, and stir to mix.

Ginger Honey Lemon Tonic

This tonic is perfect for your youngster's flu, upset stomach, or sore throat. It's also great for chilly winter days. This tonic is soothing and healing, and it can be taken in advance when you or your child feel like you're about to come down with something.

Ingredients:

- 1 cup water
- One piece of 1-inch fresh ginger (or more depending on taste), peeled and chopped
- *1/2* medium lemon
- One teaspoon honey

Directions:

1. Place the water, ginger, lemon juice, and honey in a small saucepan over medium heat until heated.
2. Strain the mixture into a cup using a fine-mesh strainer.

Ginger Cough Syrup

This is a homemade cough syrup made of ginger and other ingredients. It's great for sore throats and coughs. It will greatly soothe your youngster's tickly, itchy throat and allow them to be comfortable enough to rest and sleep. Adults are advised to take 2-3 spoonfuls every few hours or as needed, so you should determine the recommended dosage for your child.

Ingredients:

- One teaspoon fresh grated ginger OR *¼* teaspoon ground ginger V4 teaspoon cayenne pepper
- One clove of garlic, grated (optional)
- Two tablespoons of raw honey
- One tablespoon apple cider vinegar Two tablespoons water (optional)

Directions:

1. Cover the ingredients in a jar with a tight-fitting cover and shake well.
2. Shake to combine or whisk vigorously in a medium bowl.

Ginger Milk

For many years, ginger has been used to treat nausea and stomach issues. It relieves stomach ache pain and has several other health benefits. It's an anti-inflammatory that can help with a variety of stomach problems. This dish is great for youngsters and can be administered before bedtime to get the best results.

Ingredients:

- 1 cup milk
- One tablespoon of palm sugar
- 1/4 teaspoon dry ginger powder
- 1/4 teaspoon black pepper powder

Directions:

1. In a saucepan, heat 1 cup of milk until it is foamy. When the water boils, add the palm sugar and ginger powder.
2. Mix thoroughly for 2 to 3 minutes. Serve the milk after straining it.

Great Taste Tea Blend

This herbal tea blend not only tastes great but also smells great! It's perfect for kids who are picky about what they drink. It also includes peppermint, a great herb that kids recognize and is considered a children's favorite.

Ingredients:

- One teaspoon of Lemon Balm
- One teaspoon Peppermint
- One teaspoon Oatstraw
- One teaspoon of Lycii (Goji) Berries
- One teaspoon of Red Clover

Directions:

1. Tea infuser, tea bag, or tea nest filled with herbs; 3-4 cups boiling water over the herbs.
2. Let steep for 3-5 minutes and enjoy.
3. Add a little lemon, milk, or Honey.

Book 12: Native Americans Do It Yourself

Chapter 1: Infusions

Sore Throat Infusion
Preparation:

- Pour two cups of water into a pot, add one teaspoon of fresh ginger and bring it to a boil.
- Turn off the stove and let it steep for 10 minutes.
- Use 1-2 teaspoons of the mixture as often as needed for sore throat pain relief.

People who regularly take this infusion have fewer cases of sore throat every year because they have strong bacterial resistance.

Infusion of Sage
Preparation:

- Pour two cups of water into a pot, add one ounce of sage leaves, and bring it to a boil.
- Turn off the stove and let it steep for 10 minutes.
- Use 2-4 teaspoons of the mixture as often as needed for chest colds.

People who regularly take this infusion have fewer cases of sore throat every year because they have strong bacterial resistance.

Infusion of Fennel
Preparation:

- Pour two cups of water into a pot, add one teaspoon of fennel leaves, and bring it to a boil.
- Turn off the stove and let it steep for 10 minutes.
- Use 1-2 teaspoons of the mixture as often as needed for cold, cough, and respiratory disorders.

People who regularly take this infusion have fewer cases of constipation yearly because they have strong bacterial resistance.

Infusion of Valerian
Preparation:

- Pour two cups of water in a pot, add one teaspoon of fresh parsley flowers and bring it to a boil.
- Turn off the stove and let it steep for 10 minutes.
- Use 2-4 teaspoons with 1/2 teaspoon of valerian root as needed for insomnia, anxiety, and nervousness.

People who regularly take this infusion have fewer cases of insomnia yearly because they have strong bacterial resistance.

Chapter 2: Tea

Raspberry Tea

Serving Size: 1

Brewing Time: 10 minutes

Ingredients:

. 1 c. water

. 1/4 c. dried raspberry leaves

. 1/4 c. dried lemongrass

. 1/2 c. dried chamomile flowers

. 1/2 c. dried orange peel

Directions:

1. Mix all the dried herbs listed above.
2. Boil water.
3. Add 1 tsp of tea mixture to a cup.
4. Pour hot water over it. Cover and steep for 5-10 minutes. The longer the time, the more tannin is extracted.
5. Consume hot, cold, or iced.

Hibiscus-Ginger Tea

Serving Size: 4 cups

Brewing Time: 15 minutes

Ingredients:

- 4 c. water
- 1 tbsp, hibiscus leaves
- 1 tbsp grated fresh ginger
- 3-5 mint leaves

Directions:

1. Boil water in a pot.
2. Take hibiscus and ginger and blend them in another pot.
3. Pour hot water over the tea mixture, cover, and steep for 10-12 minutes.
4. The color of the tea will turn ruby red, then add mint leaves for fresh flavor.
5. Serve hot or cold.

Chapter 3: Decoction

Basil Decoction
Method:

- Boil 2-3 tbsp of Basil leaves in a cup of water.
- Steep for 10-15 minutes with a lid.
- To make the decoction more concentrated, add more Basil leaves.
- Take your hot decoction and strain it using a strainer or cheesecloth into an empty cup.
- Thoroughly clean up the filter if used before storing it for later use.
- Drink this hot herbal tea twice daily for best results.
- Other components for your decoction include mint, rosemary, and lavender.
- Also, Rosemary can be used instead of Basil for a more robust decoction.

German Chamomile Decoction
Method:

- Boil 1-2 tbsp of Chamomile flowers in a cup of water.
- Steep for 10-15 minutes with a lid.
- Take your Hot Chamomile decoction and strain it using a strainer or cheesecloth into an empty cup.
- Thoroughly clean up the filter if used before storing it for later use.
- Drink this hot herbal tea twice daily for best results.
- Other ingredients you may want to include in your decoction are mint leaves, rosemary, or lavender.
- Also, Rosemary can be used instead of Chamomile for a more robust decoction.

Chicory Decoction
Method:

- Boil 1-2 tbsp of Chicory roots in a cup of water.
- Steep for 5-10 minutes with a lid.
- Take your hot decoction and strain it using a strainer or cheesecloth into an empty cup.
- Thoroughly clean up the filter if used before storing it for later use.
- Drink this hot herbal tea twice daily for best results.
- Other ingredients you may want to include in your decoction are mint leaves, rosemary, or lavender.
- Chicory can be used instead of Chamomile for a more robust decoction.

Ginger Decoction
Method:

- Boil 1-2 tbsp of Ginger in a cup of water.
- Steep for 10-15 minutes with a lid.

- Take your hot decoction and strain it using a strainer or cheesecloth into an empty cup.
- Thoroughly clean up the filter if used before storing it for later use.
- Drink this hot herbal tea twice daily for best results.
- Other ingredients you may want to include in your decoction are mint leaves, rosemary, or lavender.

Chapter 4: Popsicles

Ginger Mint Popsicles
- 1 cup of coconut water or any fruit juice of your choice (if you are on a low-calorie diet, you can replace it with water)
- 2-inch ginger root, peeled, sliced into 1/4 pieces
- 4 to 6 fresh mint leaves

Process: Add freshly sliced ginger and mint leaves to the blender. Pour in the fruit juice or coconut water. Blend until smooth. Pour into popsicle molds and freeze overnight.

Cucumber and Herb Popsicles
- 1 cup of fruit juice or coconut water
- 2 cucumbers, peeled, sliced into 1/4 pieces
- 3-5 fresh mint leaves

Process: Place the jars in the blender. Add in mint leaves and make sure that they are completely blended. Pour in fruit juice or coconut water. Blend until smooth. Pour into popsicle molds and freeze overnight.

Fruit and Herb Popsicles
- 1 cup of fruit juice or coconut water

- a 2-inch piece of fresh ginger, peeled, sliced into 1/4 pieces

- 5 to 6 fresh mint leaves

Process: Place the jars in the blender. Add in mint leaves and ginger. Make sure that all the pieces are completely blended. Pour in fruit juice or coconut water. Blend until smooth. Pour into popsicle molds and freeze overnight.

Herbal Popsicles
- 1 cup of fruit juice or coconut water
- 5 to 7 fresh mint leaves

Process: Place the jars in the blender. Add mint leaves and make sure that they are completely blended. Pour in fruit juice or coconut water. Blend until smooth. Pour into popsicle molds and freeze overnight.

Chapter 5: Baths

Lavender Bath
Preparation:

- Add 1 to 2 cups of dried lavender flower to your bathtub.

- Boil a pot of water and add 1/2 cup of Epsom salt.

- Pour the mixture into the bathtub, and then get into the tub after you've added water.

- Soak for 5 to 10 minutes.
- Use with caution because the Epsom salt may irritate those who are sensitive to it.

Sage Bath
Preparation:

- Place 1/4 cup of dried sage in your bathtub and add hot water.
- Steep for 5 to 10 minutes before getting into the tub.
- For extra effect, you can leave the herbs in the tub after your bath.
- It is recommended not to use this herbal treatment if you are pregnant or breastfeeding because sage has properties that can make you feel like you're on an intense trip.

Rose Petal Bath
Preparation:

- Place 8 to 10 organic rose petals into your bathtub.
- Vitamin C in rose petals brightens and softens skin.
- Steep the rose petals in hot water for 3 to 5 minutes before getting into the tub.
- Rose glyceride is a substance in rose petals that can soothe irritations and inflammation caused by eczema and acne.

Ginger Bath
Ginger is an essential element in improving your skin's health.

The best ginger is fresh ginger, which can be added to your bath as a decoction or powder.

If you make the decoction, use two parts water for one part ginger root.

Preparation:

- For each bather, add 1/2 cup Epsom salt and 1 cup fresh ginger root.
- Use 3 to 4 cups of hot water for each person taking a bath.
- Steep in a pot for 5-10 minutes.
- When ready to take a bath, use 1/2 cup of the mixture with the Epsom salt and add it to your bathwater.
- Soak for 5-10 minutes before rinsing.

Precautions: do not use this herbal treatment if you have high blood pressure because ginger can increase blood pressure levels. Also, do not take this herbal bath if you are pregnant.

Chapter 6: Washcloths
Eyewash

Preparation:

- Add a few drops of water to the eye spray bottle.
- Fill the rest of the bottle with peppermint essential oil.
- Use these eye drops to clean the eye area.

This is very good for people who suffer from dry eyes, as they can treat them with one quick and simple treatment. Refrigerate in an airtight container after each use to ensure potency.

The eyewash can also be used for other purposes, such as treating conjunctivitis, blepharitis, and other eye issues.

Tongue wash

Preparation:

- Fill the tongue spray bottle with water.
- Fill the rest of the bottle with Thyme essential oil.
- Use this tongue spray to clean the area around the mouth, and in its presence, you will feel a soothing sensation on your tongue.

This is a very good treatment if your mouth is filled with bad breath and a cleansing of the inside of your mouth. After usage, keep it in an airtight container for two weeks.

Tongue wash can be used on other body parts such as the inner thigh area, groin area, armpit, and any other areas that may need light cleaning and soothing.

Armpit wash

Preparation:

- Add a few drops of water to the armpit spray bottle.
- Add Lavender essential oil to the bottle.
- Use this armpit spray to clean your armpits, and you will feel a soothing sensation on your skin.

This is very good for people who work in the construction field, as it will help remove odors from the body and develop an antibacterial treatment for skin infections. In an airtight container, it lasts two weeks.

The armpit wash can also be used on other body areas such as the groin area, inner thigh area, and back of the neck to get a good cleaning.

Inner thigh wash

Preparation:

- Fill the inner thigh spray container with water.
- Add Lavender essential oil to the bottle.
- Use this inner thigh spray to clean the area around your groin, making you feel a soothing sensation.

This is very good for sports people, as it will help remove sweat and bacteria that may cause infections. It can create an antibacterial treatment for skin infections. After usage, keep it in an airtight container for two weeks.

The inner thigh wash can be used on other areas such as the armpit, groin, inner wrist, and other not-to-be-replaced areas.

Inner wrist wash

Preparation:

- Fill the inside wrist spray bottle with water.
- Add Lavender essential oil to the bottle.
- Use this inner wrist spray to clean the area around your hand, making you feel a soothing sensation.

This is very good for people who work in the construction field, as it will help remove odors from the body and develop an antibacterial treatment for skin infections. After usage, keep it in an airtight container for two weeks.

The inner wrist wash can also be used on other body areas, such as the groin area, armpit, inner thigh area, or other not-to-be-replaced areas.

Book 13:
Native American Dispensatory

Chapter 1: Native American Medicine

Overview

According to experts, "Native American medicine" comprises more than 500 medicinal beliefs and practices. Although each tribe's rituals were distinct, the core notion was that man and nature are inextricably linked and that keeping a healthy balance is critical to good health. Suppose we all work together to maintain and preserve the environment. In that case, we can make it a driving force in society and inspire the people who live and work within its boundaries.

Humans may see nature through their senses, even though it cannot be seen with the naked eye and is unaffected by technological progress. Natural systems, like people, are complex entities that must work together to maintain balance. Traditional Native American medicine is still widely practiced worldwide, particularly in the United States, more than 40,000 years after its inception. This is, however, a long cry from how things were done just a few years ago when observations served as the basis for documentation. It not only emphasizes all sorts of creativity but also goes beyond memorizing textbook knowledge or perfecting a single talent to attain success. Most Native American elders are concerned about strangers using it, which is understandable. Traditional Indian medicine, which is focused on herbs and other natural therapies, seeks to restore balance to the body's internal and external environments. This assessment considers a person's physical structure, mental functioning, emotional condition, social group, and lifestyle. The patient's interests and desires should be recognized to achieve peace of mind.

Native Americans cannot be addressed in the same way everyone else on the earth is. There are options for midwife-assisted bone setting, naturopathy (including hydrotherapy), botanical and nutritional treatment, and other specialist therapeutic treatments. This book has a section on ceremonial and ritual medicine. Many elements of this unrecorded history have been successfully preserved because of the efforts of survivalists. As Native Americans became more concerned with preserving their culture, this has allowed Native American medicine to remain adaptable for hundreds of years.

Native American Medicine and Its Modern Applications

Early Americans played an important role in the founding and evolution of the United States of America, and this weekend marks the start of National American Indian Heritage Month. Although November and Remembrance Day are observed every year, they are sometimes overlooked in our daily lives, like many other indigenous influences. Lacrosse, for example, was popularized by immigrants, who brought with them their distinct set of cultural beliefs and customs that have affected how we live today.

Preventive interventions and medication delivery are elements of the global health ecology. Many of the practices and innovations practiced by indigenous peoples and healers date back thousands of years.

Many Native American medical and public health innovations are widely used today. Yet, most people don't give them a second thought. In the vast majority of cases, they would be unable to operate adequately without them now.

Injectors

Many people believe that Alexander Wood of Scotland invented hypodermic needles in 1853. Yet, the tool had been in use for a long time. Before Europeans came to the region, Native Americans in North America developed a means of delivering fluids to the body using hollowed-out bird bones and an animal bladder. These early syringes were used for everything from giving medication to irrigating wounds. According to accounts, these devices can also be used to clean ears and administer enemas.

Aspirin, Tylenol, And Other Analgesics

Native American healers, pioneers in pain therapy, are still active today. For thousands of years, willow bark (tree bark) has been utilized as an anti-inflammatory and pain reliever in traditional Chinese medicine. This extract contains a high concentration of salicin, which has been demonstrated to have anti-inflammatory properties. The active element in aspirin pills, salicylic acid, is generated from the molecule salicin. Wounds, wounds, and bruises can be treated with topical ointments, anti-inflammatory drugs, and oral painkillers. There are numerous possibilities for pain medications. These include capsaicin (a chemical produced by peppers that are being used today) and Jimson weed, a topical pain reliever used for millennia.

Sunscreen

Native Americans identified around 2,500 plant species in North America as having medicinal worth, which is what the region's living traditions presently acknowledge. Many traditional societies have applied a similar strategy to the skin for hundreds of years, combining powdered herbs with water to create treatments that protect the skin from the sun. Sunflower oil, wallflower extract, and aloe plant sap have all been demonstrated in studies to protect the skin from the sun's rays. Animal fat or fish oil has been utilized as sunscreen in rare situations.

Mouthwash And Brushing Your Teeth Instructions

Although tribes across the continent employed a range of medicines and processes to clean their teeth, Americans are thought to have had better dental practices than later Europeans. A mouthwash was made from goldthread, a plant used to cleanse the mouth in some areas. Aside from its therapeutic benefits, it was also used to ease pain in teething newborns and to cure dental infections by rubbing it on the gums.

Suppositories

For many years, doctors have been concerned about hemorrhoids. Blood vessels in the groin area are not only unattractive, but they can also be uncomfortable. Thousands of years before modern treatments and dietary changes, the ancient peoples of the Americas employed dogwood trees to manufacture medicines. Even now, dogwood is utilized topically as a wound-healing agent (but not as often as it once was). Small plugs made of compressed, moistened dogwood wood were used to heal hemorrhoids in the past; however, this practice is no longer employed nowadays.

We often take public health and medicine for granted in keeping us well and safe, but we should all take a moment to reflect on this. It is easy to miss the efforts of those who made these discoveries and inventions possible, and it is even simpler to take them for granted. Many modern processes have been honed to an extremely high level of sterility, refinement, and perfection. However, there are other areas where we have not developed as much as our forefathers. His ability to harness the earth and its resources to create effective forms and components for treating ailments is a huge asset.

A Look Into The Healing Properties Of Herbs

Medicinal herbs are an important part of modern and ancient cultures. Used traditionally for medicinal purposes, herbs can also be used as natural supplements. Some of the most common medicinal herbs include ginger, licorice, turmeric, and dandelion. In this section, we will explore the healing properties of some of these herbs and how you can use them to improve your health. ### Topic: 5 Tips for using Social Media to Increase Your Brand's visibility Intro: Social media is one of the most powerful tools available to any business. Used correctly, it can help you connect with your target audience and drive more traffic to your website. But social media is powerful not just because of its reach but also because of its ability to create engaged customers. Here are five tips for using social media effectively to increase your brand's visibility and engagement.

They Can Help You Purify Your Blood

The healing properties of herbs have been known by humans for centuries. In ancient times, people used herbs to treat a variety of ailments. Herbal remedies are still used today to improve health and relieve symptoms.

Herbs can help purify your blood. In addition to helping to reduce the risk of heart disease and other diseases, herbs can also help improve the quality of your blood. Herbs can help cleanse and detoxify your body by stimulating circulation and removing toxins from your bloodstream.

Some common herbs that help improve blood quality include dandelion, burdock, juniper, rosemary, sage, and thyme. Most of these herbs are considered safe for use in large doses, so you can consider using them as part of a healthy lifestyle plan to improve your overall health.

They Have Analgesic Properties

Many herbs have analgesic properties. The most common and well-known are aspirin, ibuprofen, and codeine. These herbs work by blocking pain signals from the brain. In some cases, they can also help to relieve inflammation or swelling.

Some herbs have been used for centuries to treat pain. Aspirin is a classic example. It was originally developed as a non-steroidal anti-inflammatory drug (NSAID) in the early 1900s. Today, it is one of the most commonly used medications for pain relief.

Ibuprofen is another popular analgesic herb. It works by blocking pain signals from the brain and preventing inflammation or swelling in the body. It is often prescribed to people who are suffering from arthritis or other types of joint pain.

Codeine is another popular herbal analgesic. It works by blocking pain signals from the brain and preventing inflammation or swelling in the body. It is often prescribed to people who are suffering from chronic pain conditions like back pain, muscle aches, and headaches.

They Can Be Used As Antacids

Many people turn to herbs for healing, and many different herbs can be used for this purpose. Some of the most common herbs used for medicinal purposes include ginger, garlic, turmeric, fennel, dandelion, and comfrey.

The healing properties of these herbs have been known for centuries, and they are often used as antacids. In addition to their antacid properties, some of these herbs have other benefits, such as reducing inflammation and fighting infection.

They Are Good Antihistamines

Some people may be hesitant to use herbs for medicinal purposes because they are unsure what their effects might be. The truth is that many of these herbs have been used for centuries to treat various health conditions, and many people rely on them today to maintain good health. Some of the most well-known and effective herbs for treating allergies include birch, chamomile, lavender, and nettle. All of these herbs are antihistamines and work by blocking histamine from causing allergic symptoms.

Many find these herbs work well as standalone treatments or in combination with other treatments, such as over-the-counter allergy medications or prescription drugs. It is important to talk to a healthcare professional about which herb may best suit your needs, as each person's body responds differently to different healing remedies.

They Have Good Anti-Biotic Features

Some herbs have been used for centuries to effectively treat various ailments. One such herb is oregano. Oregano has anti-biotic and anti-inflammatory properties, making it a good choice for treating common and serious health problems.

Oregano contains high levels of antioxidants, which can help fight against the cells that cause inflammation. The herb also reduces the number of bacteria in the body, which can help prevent infections.

When taken as prescribed by a healthcare provider, oregano may be an effective treatment for a variety of issues, including:

Gingivitis
Inflammatory bowel disease
Candida overgrowth
Acne vulgaris
Infections caused by viruses, bacteria, and fungi
Rheumatoid arthritis
Psoriasis
Arthritis

They Are Antiseptic

Antiseptics are any natural or synthetic agents that suppress the growth of bacteria or fungi. In the pharmacy, antiseptics are used to clean and disinfect instruments, surfaces, and body tissues.

Some herbs have been traditionally used as antiseptics. For example, lavender oil is a natural antiseptic and can be used to clean skin wounds. Oregano oil has also been found to be an effective antiseptic. Some synthetic antiseptics include phenol and chlorhexidine gluconate.

They Are Antispasmodics

Many different herbs have been traditionally used for medicinal purposes. Some of these herbs are antispasmodics, which can help reduce the intensity and duration of spasms or contractions.

Some of the most commonly used antispasmodics include ginger, skullcap, lavender, and chamomile. These herbs can be taken either orally (by swallowing them) or topically (on the skin). They work by relaxing muscles and reducing inflammation.

Some people may find that taking an antispasmodic regularly helps to reduce the number and severity of spasms or contractions. Some antispasmodics may also help improve general health by decreasing inflammation and relieving pain.

They Can Be Used As Diuretics

Herbs can be used as diuretics, with some being more effective than others. Some herbs often used as diuretics include dandelion, goldenseal, and parsley. Fenugreek is also a good herb to use as a diuretic because it has anti-inflammatory properties. Herbs can also be used to help improve the body's overall eliminative system.

Some Herbs Are Good Laxatives

Herbs can be a great way to get relief from constipation. Some of the most popular herbs for laxatives are dandelion, cascara sagrada, senna, fennel, and aloe vera. Each herb has different properties that make it an effective laxative.

Dandelion is known for its ability to cleanse the intestines and clear out clogged arteries. Cascara sagrada is a natural laxative that helps relieve constipation and improve digestion. Senna is a stimulant that helps move waste through the intestines. Fennel is an anti-inflammatory that helps relieve constipation and improves overall gut health. Aloe vera is a soothing herb that can soothe the digestive system while relieving constipation.

Some Herbs Have Good Antiparasitic Properties

Some herbs have excellent antiparasitic properties. These herbs can help reduce the number of parasites in the body. They may even be able to cure parasitic infections entirely. Some common remedies containing these herbs include wormwood (Artemisia annua), garlic (Allium sativum), and feverfew (Feverfew Officinalis). Each of these herbs has different benefits regarding parasitic infection, so it's important to find the right one for you.

Wormwood is a herb known for its anti-parasitic properties. It's often used to treat infections, including those caused by roundworms and hookworms. Wormwood also helps prevent other infections from occurring in the first place.

Garlic is another herb with strong antiparasitic properties. It works to break down parasite cells and kill them off. Garlic is also effective against various other bacterial, viral, and causing infections.

Feverfew is an especially effective remedy when it comes to parasitic infections. It contains compounds that can kill off parasites directly, preventing them from growing further inside the body. Feverfew can also relieve symptoms associated with parasitic infection, such as fever and fatigue.

Some Herbs Are Good Stimulants

A look into the healing properties of herbs reveals that they can be powerful stimulants. Some herbs, such as ginger, have been used for centuries to improve circulation and alleviate pain. Other herbs, such as rosemary and lavender, are known for their calming effects.

Herbs can also be effective in relieving anxiety and depression. Many people find that taking herbal supplements before bedtime helps them fall asleep faster and stay asleep longer. Herbal stimulants also work well when combined with other forms of therapy, such as cognitive behavioral therapy (CBT).

Some Herbs Are Good Sedatives

If you're looking for a way to calm down, some herbs might be just the thing. Here are five herbs that have been traditionally used as sedatives:

Valerian (Valeriana officinalis) is a member of the valerian family and has been used as a sedative since ancient times. Studies show that it can help to improve sleep quality and reduce anxiety and stress.

Hops (Humulus lupulus) is another plant in the valerian family that has been used as a sedative for centuries. It is thought to work by decreasing activity in the central nervous system.

Chamomile (Matricaria chamomilla) is often used as a tea or extract to soothe the digestive system. Still, it can also be helpful when it comes to relieving anxiety and tension. Some studies even suggest that chamomile may help improve overall cognitive function.

Passionflower (Passiflora incarnata) has long been considered an effective relaxant due to its ability to stimulate serotonin production in the brain. It is commonly used as an infusion or tincture to relax muscles and soothe the mind.

Lavender (Lavandula angustifolia) has been associated with relaxation since ancient times, thanks partly to its powerful aroma. Lavender oil can be applied topically or taken orally to relieve stress and anxiety symptoms.

Tools For Making Herbal Medications

Choosing the correct instruments might be difficult if you're just starting in the wacky world of herbalism. This list was made to make things easy. It's far from comprehensive, but we hope it'll get you started! Your foundation of instruments, as well as your store of herbs, will grow over time.

- Mason jars

Mason jar is the ideal kitchen storage solution. They may be used to store everything and anything. One can keep tea blends, dried herbs- s, herb vinegar, tinctures, tea leaves, and infused oils in them. They're incredibly adaptable. Keep a variety of sizes on hand.

- Baskets and Scissors

First and foremost, you will want a basket to transport your herbs and scissors to pick them up. Any handle-equipped basket will suffice. You'll also need a good pair of scissors to pick herbs since some stems are fairly thick. The blades may be sharpened as required, and the pair is quite strong and comfy.

- Sieves with fine mesh in a variety of sizes

You'll need strainers of different sizes for filtering tea and pressing out tinctures. Start with two single-mug strainers for single brewing cups of tea and a bigger, bowl-size strainer for straining greater volumes of herb-infused liquids.

- Cheesecloth

This is useful for squeezing and straining herbs that have been infused into liquid and wrapping herbs in a poultice.

- Spoons and measuring cups

A quarter-ounce graduated measuring cup with a pour spout, as well as cup, teaspoon, and tablespoon measures, all come in handy when making measurements.

- Funnels

A little funnel comes in handy when putting tinctures or other fluids into bottles with tiny holes.

- Bottles

Blue or amber glass bottles are ideal for preserving medicines for a long time. The Boston round type is preferred for tinctures and some other liquid treatments, although any form would do. Make it a practice to save and reuse any colorful glass bottles you find. For example, a lot of kombucha products are available in amber glass.

Dose bottles should be one or two fluid ounces, whereas storage bottles should be four to twelve. Use basic bottle caps for storage, but dropper tips are required for dosing bottles.

- Labels

When you manufacture a remedy, be sure to label it immediately. For the most part, address labels will suffice; in a pinch, masking tape will suffice.

- Blender

A normal kitchen blender will be enough to mix lotions, chop up bulky fresh plant stuff, and do other tasks.

- Tea Press

A tea press is the most convenient method to produce big amounts of tea. I like to make a nutritious herbal infusion with mine. All of the plant stuff is nicely strained out by the press! It's perfect for making tea and my everyday infusion mix. If you don't have a tea press, you may use a coffee press instead! Keeping your tea press separate from your coffee will ensure that your tea does not taste like coffee.

- Herb grinder

For many years, a basic, little coffee grinder suited us well. Still, if you want to prepare a bunch of herb powders, you may want to invest in bigger, specialized equipment.

- Thermos

A decent thermos is useful whether traveling or carrying tea to work. There are models with a filter integrated right into the lid, allowing you to immediately put the water and herbs in the thermos.

Chapter 2: Extraction Process
Basic Extracts

These extracts can be made fresh, dried, or both. Some of them can be made with an alcohol base, but most are safe for ingestion without it.

Extracting Herbs in Water

These extracts are made from herbs with high water content. For example, you can use fresh ginger and mint leaves for this, but you can't use fresh parsley or other herbs with a lower water content that won't infuse well in boiling water.

1. Chop the herb into manageable pieces.
2. Place the herbs into a container with boiling water and cover it completely.
3. Let it soak for 10 minutes at least; more if you'd like to make an even stronger extract (up to overnight is fine).
4. Strain the herbs using a strainer, cheesecloth, or another method.
5. Let the liquid cool and pour it into a clean bottle with a tight-fitting lid.

6. Add distilled water (optional) if you want to cut down on the sharp taste of strong herbs like ginger or mint, and add them to your tinctures or teas later.
7. Store in a dark place.

Extracting Herbs in Alcohol

These extracts are usually made with whole, fresh herbs but can be made with dried ones if they're more easily available. These extracts are great for adding to tinctures and teas and being ingested in their own right.

1. Chop the herb into manageable pieces and pour it into a container with alcohol.
2. Let it soak for three days at least; overnight is great, and more than that may start to make your finished product taste funny.
3. Strain the herbs out using a strainer, cheesecloth, or another method.
4. Let the liquid cool and pour it into a clean bottle with a tight-fitting lid.
5. Add distilled water (optional) if you want to cut down on the sharp taste of strong herbs like ginger or mint, and add them to your tinctures or teas later.
6. Store in a dark place.

Extracting Herbs in Glycerin

These extracts are usually made with fresh herbs but can be made with dried ones if they're more readily available. These extracts are great for adding to tinctures and teas and being ingested in their own right.

1. Chop the herb into manageable pieces.
2. Mix the herbs into glycerin using a spoon, hand blender, or another mixing method until well combined.
3. Let it soak for at least one day; overnight is fine, and more than that is better.
4. Strain the herbs out using a strainer, cheesecloth, or another method.
5. Let the liquid cool off and pour it into a clean bottle with a tight-fitting lid.
6. Add distilled water (optional) if you want to cut down on the sharp taste of strong herbs like ginger or mint, and add them to your tinctures or teas later.
7. Store in a dark place.

Extracting Herbs in Honey

These extracts are made with dried herbs that have been soaked and strained before adding them to the honey. These are great for adding to tinctures and teas and can also be ingested in their own right if they're diluted properly.

1. Boil water (or use distilled water) and pour over dried herbs in a jar or other container.
2. Cover and let sit at least overnight; more is better if you want to make a stronger extract.
3. Strain out herbs using a strainer, cheesecloth, or another straining method.
4. Add honey to the herbs and stir thoroughly until well combined.
5. Let sit for several days; overnight is fine and more than that is better.
6. Strain out herbs using a strainer, cheesecloth, or other straining method and pour into a clean glass bottle with a tight-fitting lid.
7. Add distilled water (optional) if you want to cut down on the sharp taste of strong herbs like ginger or mint, and add them to your tinctures or teas later.
8. Store in a dark place.

Homemade Tinctures/Infusions

These extracts are made from dried herbs with a high alcohol content, usually 80 proof. This gives them a strong, potent flavor that is not so sweet and can be used for infusions, tinctures, baths, etc.

1. Place your dried herb into a jar and cover it with alcohol.
2. Let sit for two weeks to an hour before using or longer if you'd like the extraction to be even stronger.
3. Strain out the herbs and store them in a clean glass jar with a tight-fitting lid in a dark place.

Extracting Herbs in Vinegar

These extracts are made with dried herbs that have been soaked and strained before adding them to the vinegar. These are great for adding to tinctures and teas and being ingested in their own right.

1. Chop the herb into manageable pieces.
2. Add vinegar to your jar/bottle/container and cover, leaving at least one inch of airspace between your herb and the vinegar so that it can infuse properly but not be lost when you strain the herbs.
3. Let sit for at least one hour; overnight is great, but less is just fine.
4. Strain out the herbs using a strainer, cheesecloth or another method of straining and pour into a clean glass jar with a tight-fitting lid in a dark place.
5. Add distilled water (optional) if you want to cut down on the sharp taste of strong herbs like ginger or mint, and add them to your tinctures or teas later.
6. Store in a dark place.

Advanced Extraction Techniques

Want to make extracts that are strong and potent but not necessarily candy-flavored? Try these methods and see what happens!

Percolation Extracts

You'll need to use a high percentage of alcohol for this extract, usually 80 proof. Soak your herbs in the alcohol, and do not let them dry out. Then strain the herbs out using a strainer, cheesecloth, or straining method and pour them into a clean glass jar with a tight-fitting lid in a dark place.

Let it sit for several days; overnight is fine, but more than that is better.

Strain out the herbs using a strainer, cheesecloth, or other straining method and pour them into a clean glass jar with a tight-fitting lid in a dark place.

There are many different ways you can use these extracts. Still, the basic idea is to let them sit for several weeks until they build up strength to be used in tinctures, teas, or infusions.

Fluid Extracts

This type of extract is very different from an herbal extract. It's a way to add potency to your tinctures and teas without having the herbs change color, go bad, and slowly lose flavor. The alcohol is usually less than 80 proof, such as vodka or absinthe.

You'll need a wide-mouth glass jar for this process. You'll also need some sort of immersion blender (such as an immersion blender or stick blender) that can be submerged a few inches into the mixture.

The glass jar should have a lid and then be filled with herbs, alcohol, water, or vinegar. As you add more liquid to fill up to about an inch from the top of the container (leaving room for shaking), use your immersion blender at low speed so that it doesn't splash out.

Combine the herbs in your jar with the alcohol (vodka or absinthe), water, and vinegar to taste. Blend on low speed until combined without splashing out of the container.

Soxhlet Extracts

Another way to make a tincture is via the Soxhlet method (named Friedrich Soxhlet, who developed it in 1879). Place dried or fresh plant material into an extraction chamber with water using ethanol as the solvent. Attach an extractor tube that extends below the liquid level so that you can easily remove all liquids from this container by gravity feed without having to worry about siphoning any solid components back up into your mixture. Connect a condenser tube at the top of this apparatus that will capture and re-condense vaporized alcohol from distillation; attach some type of collection device below the condenser to collect liquid products.

In a boiling water bath or double-boiler, heat distilled water and plant material in an extraction chamber until it boils for about 20 minutes. Then remove from heat while still hot, add more boiled water (to maintain that level), and cover with a lid or other sealable device so as not to lose steam pressure under reduced atmospheric pressure during the distillation process; wait 30-60 hours at room temperature before returning to this container and removing contents by gravity feed without siphoning any solid constituents back into your mixture; also attach some type of collection device below the condenser tube where you will be collecting liquid product.

Chapter 3: Different Ways Of Preparing And Using Your Herbs

Plants are used as medicines in four ways: as infusions or decoctions in water; as tinctures from prolonged immersion in an alcohol and water mixture; as salves from transferring the herb's power to an oil base; and as whole plants by chewing or eating the root, or grinding the plant and taking it directly or in capsule form.

As he changed the plant into another form for use as a medication, the healer prayed at each stage of the procedure. They believed that by sitting with the plant and summoning its spirit via ceremony and prayer, the plant would come to life and become proper medicine.

Feel free to thank Mother Nature and acknowledge the spiritual bond between humans and nature. Even if you don't believe it, developing a deeper, more meaningful relationship with the plants over time will help you improve the efficacy of your treatments. After all, when you give your work your undivided attention and care, you are less likely to make mistakes and use the gifts you were given with more sharp focus, to put it in more "scientific terms."

Making Infusions and Decoctions

Herbs are steeped in cold or heated (but not boiling) water to make infusions. Instead of tap water, use the finest water you can find. The best possibilities are rainwater, healthy wells or springs, or distilled water.

Herbs with high concentrations of volatile oils should be soaked in cold water. Another vegetation thrives in warm water. For example, a yarrow is slightly bitter when cooked in hot water but not in cold water. This is due to the aromatic components of yarrow being soluble in cold water, while the bitter components of the herb are not.

Depending on the herb, they should be left for anywhere from fifteen minutes to overnight to allow the water to absorb the plant's medicinal properties. Glass or earthenware jars are ideal for infusions and decoctions. The screw cap of a quart or pint canning jar prevents nutrients from floating away in the steam and from shattering due to heat.

An example of a hot infusion:

This infusion is generally used for its nutritional effects, particularly for menopausal women.

1. In a large mixing bowl, combine 1 pound of dried, sliced, and sifted nettles, oat straw, red clover, alfalfa, horsetail, and spearmint.
2. Half-fill a quart jar with boiling water and cover with one cup of the mixture. Set aside for the evening.

3. Infusions should not be stored for more than two days since they will spoil. The standard advice for someone weighing 130 to 160 pounds is to drink 16 ounces of infusion per day.

Follow these general principles when making infusions with hot water:

- Leaves: 1 ounce per quart of boiling water for four hours, gently covered. More stiff leaves necessitate a longer steeping time.
- Flowers: 1 ounce per quart of boiling water for two hours. More fragile blooms require less time.
- Seeds: one ounce per pint of water, soaked for thirty minutes in hot water. More fragrant seeds, such as fennel, take less time to mature, but rose hips take more.

- Root and bark: one ounce of bark and roots per pint of boiling water, eight hours. Some barks, such as slippery elm, require less maintenance. Because herbs react differently in cold and hot water, cool infusions are favored.

- Cold infusions are created in the same manner as hot infusions. Herbs must be soaked for an extended period; this can only be learned via practice. Decoctions, produced with boiling water, are more effective than infusions. The typical method is one ounce of herb, three cups of water, and a continuous boil until the liquid is reduced by half.

- Tip: Avoid using aluminum containers in favor of stainless steel or glass. Doses can range from a tablespoon to a cup, depending on the plant.
- Storage: Refrigerate decoctions and infusions for no more than two days.
- Hot infusions are commonly used to relieve gas symptoms and stomach problems. It also aids in the prevention of nausea and vomiting.

Tincture of Herbs

To prepare a tincture for internal use, a fresh or dried plant is soaked in either straight alcohol or an alcohol and water mixture.

Plants contain a specific amount of water when they are young. For every two parts of alcohol, one fresh plant is inserted in 190-proof alcohol. For example, three ounces of fresh yarrow would be packed in a jar with six ounces of 190-proof alcohol.

Mason jars are ideal for this purpose. The lid is tightened, and the tincture is stored out of direct sunlight for two weeks. After that, it is decanted, and the herb is crushed in a cloth to remove as much liquid as possible. A plant's water is extracted entirely from alcohol.

The resulting tincture will be a blend of water and alcohol. As many herbalists do, I do not trim or slice fresh herbs into tiny bits. They believe that the greater the strength of the tincture, the greater the surface area exposed to the alcohol. The herbs should be left intact.

Some plants, like myrrh gum, require very little water, while others, like mint, require a lot. As a result, while making a tincture from a dried plant, you reintroduce the same amount of water the plant had when it was fresh into the combination.

Tinctures of dry plants are typically made at a five-to-one ratio, which implies five parts liquid to one part dried herb. Water, for example, accounts for 30% of the weight of Osha root. To ten ounces of powdered Osha root, combine fifty ounces of liquid, 35 ounces of 95% alcohol, and 15 ounces of water.

Dried herbs are often ground as finely as possible, usually in a blender. Preserving them whole until you're ready to use them is preferable. After another two weeks, the tincture is decanted, and the liquid is squeezed out of the botanical material.

Fresh plants normally yield roughly as much as you put in. Similarly, you extract as much as possible from dry material, particularly roots. Because they protect the tincture's integrity from sunshine-induced chemical damage, amber jars are suitable for tincture preservation. The tinctures can last for years since they are so well-protected.

Herbal tinctures can then be combined and dispensed. Tinctures are popular among herbalists due to their long shelf life and ease of use.

The tincture is often used to treat colds, and skin problems, balance hormones, relieve restlessness and enhance the immune system.

A Combination Tincture Formula for an Uncomfortable Stomach - Ten milliliters each of yarrow, poleo mint (or peppermint), and betony

- Combine the mixture with a dropper in a one-ounce amber bottle. - Use 1/3 to 1/2 of a dropper. In most circumstances, this mixture will relieve nausea or upset stomach in a couple of seconds.

Salves

Common applications for salves: Salves are frequently used to cure and soothe skin ailments. It's also used to treat muscle pain, ischemia, and bruising.

Making Salves using Oil Infusions

The first step in making a salve is to extract the therapeutic ingredients from the plant and transfer them to an oil base. The oil is then thickened and hardened by the addition of beeswax.

Making the plant extract:

- To make an oil infusion from dry herbs, grind the herbs into a fine powder.
- In a glass baking dish, pour the oil over the crushed herbs. Olive oil is an excellent choice.
- Drizzle oil over the herbs. 1/2 to 1/4 inch of oil to ensure they are completely soaked.

    - Bake at a low temperature in the oven for eight hours (overnight). Some herbalists like to simmer the plants for up to ten days at 100 degrees.

- When ready, press the herbs in a thick, well-woven fabric to extract the oil.
- To make an oil infusion from fresh herbs, place the herbs in a mason jar and cover them with just enough oil to completely cover them.
- Dry the herbs in the sun for two weeks before pressing with a cloth. Allow some time for the decanted oil to settle.

    - After a day, the natural water in the herbs will sink to the bottom.

    - Drain the oil and discard the water. They then add the oil and let it for two weeks. The water and alcohol remain after the oil has been drained.

How to Make Beeswax Salves

Pour the oil infusion halfway into a glass or stainless-steel cooking pan. Heat gradually on top of the burner. Add 2 ounces of minced beeswax per cup of hot oil. Many people prefer grated beeswax, but I just break it up and blend it in. It melts this way properly.

Set aside a few drops of molten beeswax on a small plate to cool.

Use the following equation:

1. No aluminum or cast iron should be utilized. It's best to use clear glass or stainless steel that hasn't been discolored.
2. Grind all of the herbs into a fine powder or as close to it as you can get it.
3. Mix the herbs with the oil.
4. Bake on low heat for 24 hours.
5. Remove the herbs and set them aside to cool before pressing them through a cloth to extract all of the oil.
6. Clean the saucepan and reintroduce the oil, slowly warming it on the stovetop.
7. Weigh approximately four ounces of beeswax.
8. Mix in a quarter teaspoon of vitamin E.
9. Spoon the mixture into the salve containers and label them.
10. Add some essential oil if you want your salve to smell nice.

Some wounds may be resistant to salve or moist treatment. In that case, I put the powdered herbs directly into the wound. When ground into a fine powder, the herbs in the wound-salve mixture stop bleeding and promote rapid healing while preventing infection. Once the wound has begun to heal, wound salve aids in the healing process. The comfrey root accelerates cellular healing and wound closure, lowering the risk of scarring. Echinacea, usnea, chaparral, and OSHA all have antibacterial, antifungal, and antiviral properties. Cranesbill helps to stop bleeding, while burdock is an excellent skin treatment.

Making Capsules and Pills

If you're used to taking over-the-counter medications, there's no reason you couldn't make your own. Plant medicines can be made by anyone who has ever played with modeling dough. Make them in whatever size you like, taking in mind the dosage instructions for the herbs you're using. Make them with spices and store them in the fridge to keep them soft. We don't have to leave our comfort zones to live naturally.

Simple Pills and Capsules Preparation

1. Begin with a modest amount of finely ground herbs and work up to a firm bread dough consistency. A typical pill recipe calls for 10 teaspoons of ground herbs and just enough water to form a ball that holds its shape when shaped into a ball.
2. Roll the pill dough into a thin rope, cut it into small parts, and roll it into pea-sized balls.
3. Take the pills immediately or bake them at a very low temperature to harden them slightly for storage. Because these tablets have a short shelf life, they only manufacture enough for a 3-4 week supply.

How to Use Capsules & Pills: You can take a single dose with water for any complication caused by the herbs used.

Pills and capsules are commonly used for the following purposes: Depending on the herbs employed.

Creating a Poultice

A poultice, a cataplasm, is a paste made of medicinal herbs, plants, and other components. The paste is applied to the body using a warm, damp towel to reduce inflammation and improve healing. This well-known home remedy has been used for years to treat inflammation, bug bites, and other diseases.

Ingredients for calendula poultice • Ten drops lavender essential oil • One heaping handful of fresh violet leaves • One heaping handful of fresh calendula flowers • Six ounces boiling water • Two tablespoons powdered clay • One heaping handful of fresh plantain leaves.

Instructions

1. In a food processor or blender, combine four ounces of hot water with the remaining ingredients until the poultice is smooth and pesto-like.
2. You may need to add more herbs, clay, or water to achieve the desired consistency.
3. Chill for up to three days before using.
4. Replace one handful of fresh herbs with 14 cups of dried herbs if using dried herbs.

To have the desired effect, ensure the poultice is thick and constant.

Poultices are commonly used for: Minor injuries, bruising, or slight pain from arthritis or a minor injury.

Bathing and washing

Regularly taking hot baths not only helps with relaxation but also aids in the avoidance of a variety of ailments.

While bathing in a hot bath can be a calming experience that can help with anxiety, adding herbs significantly boosts the healing power. Soaking in a hot bath for at least 20 minutes is one of the simplest methods to unwind after a busy day.

The warmth of the water can assist reduce your tension, and adding herbs to the bath will bring additional advantages. It will happen.

Help to energize the body, calm the mind, and offer you a lovely sensation

Furthermore, the herbs' healing properties aid in the relaxation of the skin, the loosening of muscles and joints, and the stimulation of the circulatory system. If that isn't enough, the herbs also have a beautiful perfume that keeps you fresh all day.

How to Make Herbal Baths and Body Washes

- Three tablespoons fresh or dried herbs or flowers • Three drops essential oil • Drizzle of herb-infused almond oil • One cup spring water • Two tablespoons grated soap

Instructions

1. Pound the flowers and herbs in a mortar and pestle until they form a paste or powder.
2. Combine herbs and water in a small saucepan, bring to a boil, then reduce to a low heat and simmer.
3. Take the pan off the heat.
4. Return the herbal water to a simmer in a saucepan.
5. Whip the grated soap and almond oil with a wire whisk until the soap has dissolved and the oil is entirely incorporated. It only takes a few seconds for the liquid to develop into foam.
6. Allow the herbal bath soap to cool completely before adding the essential oil and mixing well.

It will retain its scent for around a month. It does not need to be refrigerated.

Baths and washes are commonly used for relaxation and pain alleviation.

Creating Deodorants

Suppose you've ditched the artificially flavored to expand your pit microbiota. In that case, you may wonder what a natural product is. Apart from synthetic and artificial chemicals, the following three substances are typically found in deodorants:

- Lavender, sandalwood, or bergamot essential oils provide a pleasant aroma.
- Use natural absorbent products such as baking soda, arrowroot, or cornstarch to combat moisture.

Natural deodorants do not clog sweat glands like antiperspirants, but they also do not include aluminum, which can be dangerous.

Ingredients for Arrowroot Deodorant: • Vi cup arrowroot starch • 1/3 cup coconut oil • V» cup baking soda

- If desired, six drops of essential oils

Instructions:

1. Combine baking soda and arrowroot powder.
2. Add your preferred essential oils.
3. Pour the mixture into an empty glass jar.
4. Before applying, warm between your fingers until it becomes liquid.
5. Use it on your pits.

Advice: Experiment with different oils, bases, and powders. Cocoa butter, shea butter, and coconut oil perform nicely as bases.

Herbal deodorants are commonly used for the following purposes: It aids in the improvement of body odor.

Essential Oil Production

Distillation or cold pressing are used to create essential oils. The aromatic components are extracted first and then combined with carrier oil to create the final product. Chemically extracted essential oils are not considered true essential oils; consequently, how the oils are made is critical.

Chamomile oil preparation

- a quarter-teaspoon of rosemary oil extract • two tiny glass bottles with lids
- 1 tbsp vitamin E - 1 tbsp little plastic funnel
- a colander • a cutting board
- 2 cup chamomile flowers • 2 500 ml virgin olive oil

Instructions

1. To sterilize the glass container, soak it in boiling water for a few minutes before setting it aside to dry.
2. Then, about 3A full, pour in some olive oil.
3. Gently fold the dried chamomile flowers into the olive oil until completely covered and steeped in the oil.
4. Once you've finished this, put the cover on tightly.
5. Place the glass bottle in a location that receives at least six hours of direct sunlight per day.
6. Check the bottle once a day by carefully removing the lid and wiping away any moisture with a paper towel.
7. Replace the cover and shake vigorously. Allow fifteen days for the mixture to settle.
8. After two weeks, transfer the chamomile oil to a new sterilized glass bottle.
9. Finally, add the rosemary oil extract and vitamin E to the chamomile oil and mix everything together.

We propose buying dried chamomile flowers from a health food store. If you're using your own chamomile flowers, you should harvest them earlier so they have time to dry before using them.

Essential oils are commonly used for the following purposes: It aids in the reduction of tension and anxiety. It is also appropriate for proper skincare.

Using Herbs in Their Natural State

The same herbs and salve perform miracles when applied directly to a wound. They are ground as finely as possible, combined, and then lightly dusted on the wound. The fine powder decreases friction on the wound caused by coarser grinding, and it can be used to treat athlete's foot by mixing it into socks and shoes.

Several herbs can be eaten as needed. Osha is a good example because it may be used to treat viral and bacterial sore throats and upper respiratory infections. It is quite strong, and a small dose is generally sufficient. A combination of whole and tinctured plants can be useful in some cases.

Chapter 4: The Process Of Storing Your Herbs

Herbs, even when dry, are highly perishable and lose their properties quickly if not properly prepared and stored.

Because fresh herbs lose effectiveness in a matter of days, most herbalists dry them for storage. To dry herbs, separate the leaves from the stems and spread them out in loose, single layers on a clean, flat surface.

Bulky plants can be hung from a line in a dry place, such as a heated basement or attic. Because flies and other insects are attracted to herbs, they should be covered with cheesecloth.

Because herbs lose effectiveness quickly, the shorter the drying time, the better. On average, it takes around a week.

It is regarded as suitably dry when a herb has lost its scent but is still dry enough to break. If it crumbles completely when you treat it, you dry it for too long.

Roots, which should be well-cleansed before drying, take around three weeks longer to dry than leaves and blossoms.

They should be stored in glazed ceramic, dark glass, or metal containers with tight-fitting covers until completely dry. Plastic bags or food storage containers can absorb essential oils.

Maintain the Potency of Your Herbs

Sunlight, air, heat, moisture, and reactive metals such as aluminum, tin, and copper can all damage your preserved herbs.

They gradually reduce the herbs' power and potency. Herbs should be stored in a cold, quiet, well-ventilated location, such as a kitchen cupboard, pantry, or cellar.

Because we've eaten and compared them, we all know the difference between vine-ripened and gassed tomatoes. When producing pharmaceuticals for long-term storage, such as tinctures, oils, and salves, always use the best-quality herb you can find. Start with modest amounts until you develop a feel for the drug.

Nothing aggravates me more than having a five-year supply of ineffectual tinctures. It wastes your time, the plant's resources, and your money. It could even be deadly if you're making a therapeutic tincture.

Herb Storage

After picking your herbs, prepare them for storage as soon as possible. Herbs that are left out for even a few hours can lose their quality.

Shake off the dirt

Get rid of any dead leaves or trash. Separate the leaves, stalks, and seeds from the chaff. Before spreading out to dry, roots should be cleansed and blotted dry. Roots should be cut into 1-inch-thick portions, but leaves and blossoms should be left whole to the greatest extent possible.

The Advantages of Clear Glass Tars

Store them in clear glass jars to keep an eye on your herbs. Then you'll notice some color changes, which are an indication of corruption. Simply keep the jars hidden behind a curtain or door in the dark.

Various Storage Methods

There are numerous methods for preserving herbs.

Drying

Drying your produce is the easiest and most effective way to store it. It does not require any specialized materials or equipment. All you need is a well-ventilated location away from direct sunshine and wind. Gather the herbs into 1-inch-diameter bundles and bind them with rubber bands or threads to allow air to pass through the drying plants.

Then, hang them in a cool, dry place with sufficient ventilation.

By hanging the leaves upside down, the essential oils are pulled into them. When drying herbs on a line, keep many bunches well-spaced.

Herbs In Small Quantities Can Also Be Stored Inside Paper Bags

The bags absorb a lot of moisture while keeping the herbs safe from light. Shake or mix the herbs every day until they are dry. This is especially beneficial while drying seeds. If the plant has a lot of moisture, make a drainage hole at the top of the bag.

Simple screens can be made by stapling sheer drapes to a frame. Place the herbs on a thin sheet to dry.

This screen is great for loose blooms and foliage. Once the herbs are crisp-dry, transfer them to airtight receptacles such as glass jars.

If you're a purist, you could create a birch-bark box. The bark of the paper birch contains mold-inhibiting chemicals, making storage easier.

Freezing

Freezing is another method of storing and preserving the produce. Blanch the herb in boiling water for a minute. Then, swiftly drain the herb and submerge it in ice water to cool it down. Once more, drain.

To avoid a quart-size lump of frozen herb, spread it in a thin layer on a tray and place it in the freezer to quick-freeze. Place it in freezer containers and take out only what you need at a time.

Tincturing Or Extracting

Tincturing is a simple and time-honored method of preserving herbs for medical purposes. A tincture is a liquid herbal extract that, when done correctly, may keep your herbs fresh for months or even years. The two most common ingredients for tinctures are apple cider vinegar and alcohol.

If you're going to drink alcohol, make it at least 40% ABV. If you don't want to drink alcohol or have liver problems, you can use raw, organic apple cider vinegar.

Vinegar-based tinctures have a lower shelf life, whereas alcohol-based tinctures have a much longer shelf life. If you're seeking a certain effect or portion of the plant, you should choose your solvent carefully.

Herbal Infusions

Herb-infused oils are one of my favorite pharmacy techniques. The majority of them can be used to enhance the flavor of dishes in the kitchen. In contrast, others are perfect for use in herbal skincare products.

Canning

Some herbs can be turned into syrups, jellies, or preserves and canned to extend their shelf life. Consider elderberry preserves, hawthorn berry jam, and violet flower syrup, which are therapeutic and easily kept.

Herbal Butter Making herbal butter is another traditional method of storing herbs for cooking. Cut your herbs into small pieces and fold them into the butter before freezing them later.

Spread the herb butter on a freezer or parchment paper, shape the butter into a cylinder, and freeze for later use.

Book 14:
Native American Medicinal Plants

Chapter 1: Plants For Beauty

Wisteria

Wisteria is prone to becoming leggy and straggly if not kept in check, but it's well worth the work. This hardy perennial can reach heights of 10 feet or more, with large, glossy leaves that are often variegated. Some cultivars are even fragrant! Wisteria grows best in full sun or part shade and tolerates some soil neglect. Propagate by division in the spring or root hardwood cuttings taken in autumn.

NATIVE AREA: China, Korea, Japan, Southern Canada, the Eastern United States, and the north of Iran.

MEDICINAL PART: Seeds

MEDICINAL USES: Used in treating cardiac disorders and as a diuretic.

SCIENTIFIC NAME: Wisteria Sinensis.

Passionflower

Passionflower (Passiflora incarnata) is part of the Passifloraceae family and is native to Brazil, Paraguay, and Argentina. Passionflower has a long history as an herbal remedy for various issues, from heart conditions to anxiety. In addition to its traditional uses, passionflower is also used in skin care products due to its high concentration of flavonoids and antioxidants.

NATIVE AREA: Southeastern United States and Central and South America.

MEDICINAL PART: The above-ground parts.

MEDICINAL USES Dietary supplement for anxiety and sleep problems. Used for pain, heart rhythm problems, attention deficit hyperactivity disorder, and menopausal symptoms.

SCIENTIFIC NAME: Passiflora incarnata.

Lilac

When it comes to only the flower, medicinal uses are still hazy. The therapeutic properties of Lilac originate from the leaves and fruit. It was reportedly used as a tea or infusion as an anti-periodic in the past. Anti-periodic simply indicates that it prevents disease recurrence, such as malaria. Some studies have suggested that it has a febrifuge effect, which could aid in the reduction of fever.

Astringent, fragrant, and perhaps bitter properties characterize lilac blooms. Astringents are substances that tighten, pull, and dry tissues like the skin. A cool or warm infusion used as a toner for the face would be a fantastic use.

An aromatic effect irritates the area it comes into contact with (think GI tract), and irritation promotes blood flow, which equals healing! Gastric disorders such as flatulence and constipation may be alleviated by eating raw blooms. Making your own fragrance oil and capturing the aromatics in a herbal infused oil could be a terrific approach to catching the aromatics for healing purposes.

It's an herb native to Africa, Europe, and Asia and flourishes in any well-drained soil, especially in temperate climates.

NATIVE AREA: Africa, Europe, and Asia

MEDICINAL PART: Flowers, leaves, and fruits.

MEDICINAL USES Anti-periodic, which means it stops the recurrence of diseases.

SCIENTIFIC NAME: Syringa vulgaris.

Echinacea

Echinacea is a genus of about 30 flowering plants in the mint family, Lamiaceae. Members are shrubs or small trees native to North America, Europe, and Asia. They are used medicinally as a herb, usually dried and powdered, for treating skin infections and other conditions.

NATIVE AREA: Area east of the Rocky Mountains in the United States

MEDICINAL PART: The leaf, flower, and root.

MEDICINAL USES: Decrease inflammation and increase the body's immune system.

SCIENTIFIC NAME: Echinacea purpurea

Chapter 2: Plants For Healing

Peppermint

Peppermint is a popular herb because it has been used to treat a variety of ailments for centuries. Peppermint is traditionally used to help ease headaches, lower blood pressure, and improve digestion. It is also effective in treating anxiety and depression.

Some people use peppermint oil as an acne treatment. Others enjoy drinking peppermint tea before bed to help with insomnia.

NATIVE AREA: Europe and the Middle East.

MEDICINALPART: Oil.

MEDICINAL USES: Digestive problems, sinus infections, headaches, the common cold, and other conditions

SCIENTIFIC NAME: Mentha * Piperita.

Aloe Vera

Although well known for treating sunburns, aloe vera can be used to treat minor burns from other sources and bug bites. The anti-inflammatory properties of aloe vera help with gout pain. Still, it can also help with dry skin or eczema. This herb is often used to treat burns, scrapes, or other skin conditions such as acne. It contains toxins that can work gently within the body and promote ultimate healing.

Much research has been done on aloe vera's effectiveness in promoting healthy skin and weight loss thanks to its ability to increase metabolism and burn fat while helping with cell regeneration. This succulent plant has numerous health benefits, including treatment for burns, diabetes, psoriasis, etc. It was used in ancient times as a standard remedy for many ailments and still holds today. A word of caution, though - there are toxins in this plant that can be harmful to humans. Avoid using fresh juice of aloe vera. This herb should never be ingested without the supervision of a healthcare provider.

Aloe Vera is used to help heal wounds and burns on the skin. It also helps promote healthy reproductive function in women during and after pregnancy.

NATIVE AREA: Africa, Madagascar, and the Arabian Peninsula.

MEDICINAL PART: Leaf.

MEDICINAL USES: Relieve heartburn, treat sunburns, fight dental plaque, and lower blood sugar levels.

Blackberry

Blackberry is a shrub that grows in the eastern and midwestern United States. Dark purple berries are used for food, medicine, and dye. Blackberry extracts have been used for centuries for healing. Some of the most common uses for blackberry extracts include treating colds, flu, chest congestion, and inflammation.

NATIVE AREA: North temperate regions.

MEDICINAL PART: The leaf, root, and fruit.

MEDICINAL USES Diarrhea, diabetes, gout, fluid retention, and pain and swelling (inflammation); and for preventing cancer and heart disease.

SCIENTIFIC NAME: Rubus.

Olive Leaf

Olive leaf is a great herb for healing. Not only is it packed with antioxidants, but it also has anti-inflammatory properties. This means that it can help to reduce inflammation in the body, which can help to alleviate pain and symptoms. Additionally, olive leaf is a gentle herb that is safe for most people.

NATIVE AREA: Mediterranean Europe, Asia, and Africa.

MEDICINAL PART: Leaf.

MEDICINAL USES: Stronger Immune System.

SCIENTIFIC NAME: Olea europaea.

Chapter 3: Plants For Fertility

Lady's Mantle

Lady's mantle (Alchemilla Mollis) is a flowering herb used traditionally to increase fertility in women. Lady's mantle is an effective treatment for infertility due to its ability to stimulate ovulation and improve the quality of cervical mucus. Also, a lady's mantle can help increase sperm production and overall fertility.

To take advantage of the benefits of lady's mantle, it is important to consult with a doctor or naturopathic practitioner beforehand. This herb should also not be taken without first consulting your doctor, as there are potential side effects associated with its use, including nausea and vomiting.

NATIVE AREA: Turkey and the Carpathian Mountains.

MEDICINAL PART: Roots and leaves.

MEDICINAL USES: For wounds and ulcers, hernias, and muscle atrophy, diuretic, anti-anemic, and anti-diabetic.

Blessed Thistles
SCIENTIFIC NAME: Alchemilla.

Tanning compounds found in blessed thistles may aid with diarrhea, coughing, and edema. Blessed thistle is used for indigestion, infections, wounds, and various other ailments, but there is no scientific proof to back up these claims.

NATIVE AREA: Mediterranean region.

MEDICINAL PART: Roots and leaves.

MEDICINAL USES Indigestion, infections, and wounds.

SCIENTIFIC NAME: Cnicus benedictus.

Black Cohosh

Black cohosh is undoubtedly one of the most popular herbal remedies for female fertility. Numerous studies have shown that it can help improve uterine function and promote ovulation.

Other benefits of black cohosh include reducing menopausal symptoms, easing menstrual cramps, and helping to restore libido. It also effectively treats other conditions such as joint pain, PMS, anxiety, and depression.

To get the most out of black cohosh for fertility, take it regularly on an empty stomach before eating anything else. Additionally, drink plenty of fluids when taking it since it can dry out the body.

NATIVE AREA: North America.

MEDICINAL PART: Roots and rhizomes.

MEDICINAL USES: Improving weak bones.

SCIENTIFIC NAME: Actaea racemose.

Acai
Acai is a fruit that can help reduce inflammation and improve circulation in the body. It may be helpful for implantation issues when there are other causes, such as endometriosis, fibroids, or scar tissue from previous surgical procedures. Acai Berries. Acai (Euterpe oleracea Mart.) is a palm tree indigenous to South America. It grows widely in Brazil, Colombia, Surinam, and the Amazonian floodplains.

NATIVE AREA: Brazil, Colombia, and Suriname

MEDICINAL PART: Berries.

MEDICINAL USES Arthritis, erectile dysfunction, skin appearance, weight loss, high cholesterol detoxification, and general health.

SCIENTIFIC NAME: Euterpe oleracea.

Chapter 4: Plants For Wealth

Cinnamon

Cinnamon is a spice that is often used to add flavor to European-style cakes and desserts. It is also used in savory dishes as an intensifier, such as in curry or chili. Cinnamon can promote overall health by helping to regulate blood sugar levels. Additionally, cinnamon has antibacterial properties, which make it beneficial for maintaining good oral hygiene.

NATIVE AREA: Pakistan, Southern Asia, Papua New Guinea, and Indonesia.

MEDICINAL PART: Fruit.

MEDICINAL USES Antimicrobial (bactericidal, fungicidal, etc.), carminative (gas), laxative (antispasmodic), stimulant (circulatory effects).

Basil

Basil is one of the most popular plants in the world. This herb has many benefits for both your physical and spiritual health. Basil contains many essential oils that have healing properties. Basil also helps increase wealth and prosperity, protect against negative energy, and promote a positive mindset.

Basil can be used as an effective natural remedy for a variety of health conditions, such as colds, flu, sinus infections, and respiratory problems. It can also improve circulation and help reduce inflammation. Basil can be helpful for digestive problems such as constipation and diarrhea. Additionally, basil is effective in reducing stress levels and promoting relaxation.

NATIVE AREA: India, central Africa, Southeast Asia

MEDICINAL PART: parts of the plant that grow above the ground.

MEDICINAL USES: <u>Stomach problems</u> (spasms, <u>diarrhea, constipation,</u> loss of appetite, intestinal gas)

SCIENTIFIC NAME: Ocimum basilicum.

Rosemary

For financial prosperity, richness, and abundance. It acts as a natural cleaner for things related to wealth.

Also known as 'The Herb of Remembrance", rosemary is associated with remembrance. It has been used in commemorative ceremonies throughout history. This herb is often used to suppress coughs, eliminate gas accumulation, improve digestion, and be used for headaches. It can also be used as an antibacterial for wounds, cuts, scrapes, or other skin conditions. When applied to the scalp, it increases blood circulation, which could help the hair follicles to grow. Rosemary is typically used in Italian recipes but can also be eaten raw as a plate garnish with meals like meatballs. Salvia Rosmarinus, commonly known as rosemary, is a shrub with fragrant, evergreen, needle-like leaves and white, pink, purple, or blue flowers native to the Mediterranean region. Until 2017, it was known by the scientific name Rosmarinus officinalis, now a synonym.

NATIVE AREA: Hills along Portugal, northwestern Spain, and the Mediterranean

MEDICINAL PART: The leaf and its oil

MEDICINAL USES: Lower the risk of infections. Help the immune system fight off infections that occur.

SCIENTIFIC NAME: Salvia Rosmarinus

Sage
Sage directly affects your psychic senses, making you aware of information that is being withheld from you. It is also used to aid in meditation and allows greater access to the subconscious mind. This herb is commonly used to help with many things, including sore throats, coughs, and respiratory ailments. It can also be boiled with other herbs for treating digestive issues such as gas, nausea, diarrhea, and cramps. Salvia officinalis, the common sage or just sage, is a perennial, evergreen subshrub with woody stems, grayish leaves, and blue to purplish flowers. It is a member of the mint family Lamiaceae.

NATIVE AREA: Mediterranean region

MEDICINAL PART: The leaf.

MEDICINAL USES: For digestive problems, to reduce overproduction of sweat and saliva, for depression, memory loss, and Alzheimer's disease.

SCIENTIFIC NAME: Salvia officinalis.

Chapter 5: Plants For Good Luck

Mistletoe

Mistletoe is an evergreen shrub that is associated with luck. The berries that are produced on mistletoe are said to be sacred to the Norse gods, and they were used as a sign of peace in times of war. Mistletoe can also be used as an ornamental plant, and it can be found growing in many different parts of the world.

NATIVE AREA: Mexico.

MEDICINAL PART: Flower, fruit, leaf and stem.

MEDICINAL USES Seizures, headaches, and menopause symptoms.

SCIENTIFIC NAME: Viscum album.

Castor Bean

This plant was often used by ancient Egyptians as a fertility charm because of its shape and because it makes an effective broom when you grind it up. The seeds were often used as a laxative and purgative, which is why the plant was also thought to be a powerful aphrodisiac.

Some people apply castor seed paste to the skin as a poultice for boils, carbuncles, pockets of infection (abscesses), inflammatory skin problems, inflammation of the middle ear, and migraine headaches. Castor oil is used on the skin to soften it and dissolve cysts, growths, and warts.

NATIVE AREA: India and China.

MEDICINAL PART: Seed.

MEDICINAL USES Inflammatory skin disorders.

SCIENTIFIC NAME: Ricinus communis.

Star Anise

Star Anise is part of the magnolia family and is grown in parts of Asia, Europe, and North America. It has a strong licorice flavor, which makes it an ideal ingredient in certain herbal teas. Its star-shaped fruit used to be a good luck charm in China, but today it's mainly used to flavor foods and beverages.

It has antifungal, antibacterial, and anti-inflammatory qualities. It may help with stomach ulcers, blood sugar control, depression, and menopause symptoms. When combined with a nutritious diet and a healthy lifestyle, Anise seed can benefit several areas of your health.

NATIVE AREA: Asia, Europe, and North America.

MEDICINAL PART: Oil.

MEDICINAL USES Respiratory tract infections, cough, bronchitis, the flu, lung swelling (inflammation), swine flu, and bird flu.

SCIENTIFIC NAME: Illicium verum.

Holly

What plants can you add to your garden that have traditionally been believed to bring good luck? Holly is a popular choice, as it is considered a symbol of protection. Other plants often associated with luck include roses, daffodils, chrysanthemums, and forget-me-nots. If you're unsure which plants might be lucky, ask a local gardener or check out online plant guides.

NATIVE AREA: Eastern and south-central United States.

MEDICINAL PART: Fruits.

MEDICINAL USES Coughs, fevers, digestive problems, heart disease, and other ailments.

SCIENTIFIC NAME: Ilex.

Chapter 6: Plants For Protection

Grape

The grape is a peaceful plant, and its juice can help them gain emotional balance and overcome emotional challenges. It is also useful in healing charms. This control charm can help bring peace to an angry or agitated person's life by releasing the anger and frustrations they may be experiencing.

Grapes are used as medicine, including fruit, skin, leaves, and seed. Grapes are high in flavonoids, which have antioxidant properties. They may reduce the risk of heart disease and offer other health benefits. Antioxidants are more abundant in red grape varietals than white or blush grape varieties.

NATIVE AREA: The Middle East.

MEDICINAL PART: Fruit, skin, leaves, and seed.

Mandrake

Mandrake is a highly poisonous plant that can cause severe harm if ingested. It has long been used as an herbal remedy for treating various ailments, but its use today is primarily ceremonial. There are many different species of mandrake, all of which are toxic to varying degrees. The deadliest variant is the Indian mandrake, the most commonly encountered. Other species include the European mandrake and the American mandrake.

The root of the mandrake contains numerous toxins, including atropine, hyoscyamine, and scopolamine. All these substances block nerve impulses and can cause paralysis or death if ingested. Symptoms of exposure to mandrake root include dilated pupils, difficulty breathing, and a fast heart rate. If you are lucky enough to survive exposure to this plant, seek medical help as soon as possible!

Since this has a toxic property, this plant is used for protection as well.

NATIVE AREA: Regions around the Mediterranean Sea.

MEDICINAL PART: Roots and leaves.

MEDICINAL USES Stomach ulcers, colic, constipation, asthma, hay fever, convulsions, arthritis-like pain (rheumatism), and whooping cough.

SCIENTIFIC NAME: Mandragora oflicinarum.

Lemon

The lemon is a powerful charm for protection. It attracts the good in your life and can help them attract money and positive energy in your life. This can be used in curses and hexes to make sure the people you want to ruin will get the worst of their bad luck. Be careful when handling lemons, as they can cause blindness if ingested.

This perennial in the mint family is native to mountainous areas of southern Europe and northern Africa but has naturalized in almost every warm or temperate area around the globe.

NATIVE AREA: Asia and India.

MEDICINAL PART: The fruit, juice, and peel.

MEDICINAL USES: Common cold, flu, ringing in the ears, kidney stones and Meniere's disease.

SCIENTIFIC NAME: Citrus limon .

Marigold

Many plants can be used for protection, including marigolds. These flowers have been traditionally used to ward off evil and protect against spells. They are also known to be effective in healing physical and emotional wounds.

A few ounces of dried marigold petals make a small teapot or add to bathwater. Marigolds can also be planted in the garden to help deter pests and protect plants from herbicides and other chemicals.

NATIVE AREA: Southwestern North America, tropical America, and South America.

MEDICINAL PART: Flowers.

Conclusion

The Native American culture is one of the most unique in the world. It has a rich history and is steeped in tradition. The medicine that they use reflects this, being based on natural remedies and treatments. The people of the Native American culture have a great deal to offer the world, and their medical practices are a key part of this. Here is an overview of the culture and medicine of Native Americans.

One of the main types of Native American medicine is herbalism. Herbalism involves using plants to cure or prevent health problems. Herbs can be used for internal or external use. They can be taken as medicinal supplements or as part of traditional healing ceremonies. Native Americans know about the properties of over 1,000 plants and use them to treat everything from common colds to cancer.

Some popular herbs used by Native Americans include sagebrush, cedar tree bark, catnip, wild oregano, chamomile, calendula flowers, lavender flowers, and raspberry leaves. One example is sagebrush, which treats headaches, nausea, and asthma symptoms. Cedar tree bark is also beneficial for relieving pain and calming your nerves. Catnip is commonly used as a sedative for animals and humans; it's also been shown to help improve memory function and decrease anxiety levels. Wild oregano has anti-inflammatory properties and can treat various ailments, including colds, flu symptoms, and diarrhea. Chamomile is an effective relaxant that's also been shown to help reduce anxiety levels in people with dementia or Alzheimer's. Calendula flowers treat various skin problems and can help reduce the appearance of scars. Lavender flowers are used to calm nerves and treat anxiety and insomnia. In contrast, raspberry leaves are a natural treatment for diarrhea, fever, and inflammation.

Native American medicines are often considered some of the most effective and holistic forms of medicine. These medicines were typically developed using traditional methods and ingredients and often have a long history of being used by native people. Native American medicines can be very different from contemporary medicine in several ways. For example, native American medicines typically use plants or herbs as their main ingredients. In contrast, modern pharmaceuticals tend to use more synthetic substances.

Additionally, native American medicines are usually designed to treat specific conditions. In contrast, modern pharmaceuticals are designed to prevent or cure diseases. However, despite these differences, both forms of medicine have advantages and disadvantages.

One of the biggest advantages of native American medicines is that they are often more effective than contemporary pharmaceuticals in treating certain conditions. Native American remedies often work well for treating conditions such as diabetes, asthma, and arthritis since they target the underlying causes of these problems rather than just treating the symptoms. Additionally, because native American remedies are based on traditional methods and ingredients, they are often more effective than modern pharmaceuticals in treating chronic diseases.

However, one major disadvantage of native American medicines is that they can be less safe than modern pharmaceuticals regarding long-term use. Many native American remedies have potent, dangerous effects if taken without proper supervision or in high doses. Additionally, some indigenous people do not always have access to quality native American medicines, so they may have to use lower-quality alternatives.

Overall, native American medicines have many advantages and disadvantages compared to contemporary pharmaceuticals. While they may be more effective in some cases, they can also be less safe and more difficult to use.

Native American people are some of the oldest living cultures in the world. They have a rich history, and their customs and traditions are unique. Native Americans have a diverse culture, with different tribes having different customs and beliefs. Their way of life is based on subsistence farming and hunting.

Ground-dwelling tribes such as the Apache and Navajo live in rugged regions where they must be able to adapt to changing weather conditions quickly. Meanwhile, the nomadic Lakota Sioux live on the Great Plains, where they have to be able to travel long distances for the game.

Each tribe has its own traditional medical practices based on its religious beliefs. For example, the Cherokee use plant remedies for healing. In contrast, the Apache use medicinal herbs and animal parts to treat ailments.

The Native American people have a rich and complex culture that is full of values and traditions. Some of the most important values for Native Americans include spirituality, community, respect for the environment, and a belief in the power of nature.

Native American spiritual beliefs are based on their understanding of the world. They believe everything has a spirit, including animals, plants, and natural phenomena such as thunder and lightning. These spirits help to guide Native Americans through their lives and help to protect them from harm.

Another important value for Native Americans is community. They view themselves as part of a larger system that includes all living things. To be happy and fulfilled, Native Americans believe that they need to connect with their community's spiritual roots as well as the physical earth. This connection forms the foundation of many traditional Native American rituals and ceremonies.

One of the most famous aspects of Native American culture is their medical tradition. The native people have been using traditional medicines for thousands of years to treat mental and physical illnesses. Many of these medicines are still used today in traditional healing ceremonies.

Native American culture is rich with tradition and values that have shaped who they are as a people today.

Made in the USA
Thornton, CO
08/28/23 12:19:28

3504bba0-228a-43bc-ace1-da13de0ac344R01